YOGA THERAPY ON HO
MEN

by

RASHMITHA

ABSTRACT

Background: Menstrual health is often ignored for a number of reasons, resulting in a variety of issues such as prolonged menstruation, miscarriage, pregnancy complications, and infertility. The present study is chosen in order to determine an alternative and authentic approach through yoga, to assess the effect of yoga on the on hormone levels like estrogen and Luteinizing hormone and haemoglobin in subjects with menstrual disorder and also to evaluate the quality of life in subjects with menstrual disorders.

Objectives:

- To assess the effect of yoga therapy on hormone levels like estrogen and Luteinizing hormone in subjects with menstrual disorder.
- To analyse the outcome of yoga in improving haemoglobin level.
- To evaluate the quality of life in subjects with menstrual disorder.

Methodology: 100 subjects with menstrual disorder of the age group 18 to 25 years are selected randomly for this study. They were classified into two groups, i.e experimental and control with 50 subjects each. They were further classified into two groups, heavy bleeding and scanty bleeding based on their complaint. The control group continued with normal lifestyle. The experimental group was provided selected yogic practices, six days per week for duration of one hour. Parameters such as estradiol test, luteinizing hormone test, haemoglobin test and the quality of life were measured before and after the study to obtain the data. "Paired t" test was utilized using SPSS software in the study to analyse the significance of the result statistically.

Results: The statistical analysis of estrogen hormone, luteinizing hormone and haemoglobin levels in heavy bleeding and scanty bleeding subjects of experimental groups has shown considerable improvement and balanced level of hormones when compared to the control group. Haemoglobin level improved and the symptoms of menstrual disorder reduced in experimental group subjects.

Conclusion: Based on the experimental evidences, it is concluded that the yoga Therapy helps to improve and maintain the hormone levels, haemoglobin and the quality of life of subjects with menstrual disorder.

Keywords: Menstrual disorder, Estrogen hormone, estradiol, luteinizing hormone, Haemoglobin, yoga therapy.

ACKNOWLEDGEMENT

I express my deep sense of gratitude to my respected guide Dr. K. Krishna Sharma, M.A, M.Sc., Ph.D., Chairman, Department of Human Consciousness and Yogic Sciences, Mangalore University, Mangalagangothri – 574199, for his inspiration, encouragement and guidance throughout the present research study. I am also grateful to him for training me in Yoga Therapy.

I am grateful to my parents, brother and friends for their support and encouragement. I sincerely express my gratitude towards all my teachers because of them I am here today. I thank Dr Udayakumara K and Dr Thirumaleshwara Prasada H, Yoga consultants of the Department of Human Consciousness and Yogic Sciences, Mangalore University, for their suggestions and kind support. I am thankful to Mrs. Rajitha, Typist, and Mr. Rangappa, Research Scholar, Department of Human Consciousness and Yogic Sciences for their kind help and encouragement during the present research work. I am thankful to Dr. Rekhalatha, gynaecologist, Kanachur Hospital, Mangalore for being medical expert for this work and I am also thankful to Prof. T.P.M Pakkala, for his guidance during the statistical analysis of the data. I am thankful to all the staff members of Dept. of Human Consciousness and Yogic Sciences, for their support throughout my research study period. I thank one and all who have helped me in one or the other way directly or indirectly.

(RASHMITHA)

Contents

1. INTRODUCTION 10
   1.1 Yoga: 10
   1.2 Yoga Therapy: 11
   1.3 Background of the study: 11
   1.4 Relevance of the study: 12
   1.5 Objectives of the study: 12

2. MENSTRUAL DISORDER 14
   2.1 Overview of menstrual disorder: 14
   2.2 Menstruation: 14
   2.3 Importance of menstruation: 14
   2.4 Menstrual Disorders: 15
   2.5   Prevalence of menstrual disorder: 15
   2.6 Aetiology of menstrual disorder: 15
   2.7 Types of menstrual disorder: 16
   2.8 Role of hormones: 18

3. YOGIC MANAGEMENT OF MENSTRUAL DISORDER: 20
   3.1 Rajodarsana/ Menstruation 20
   3.1.1 Tridosha theory: 23
   3.1.2 Panchakosha theory: 24
   3.1.3 Sadvimshati tattva theory: 26
   3.1.4 Principles and approach of yoga therapy: 27
   3.2 Yoga therapy for menstrual disorders: 28
   3.2.1   Lifestyle: 28
   3.2.2   Asana: 28
   3.2.3 Physiological contributions of asana: 29
   3.2.4   Pranayama: 31
   3.2.5   Physiological contributions of Pranayama: 32
   3.2.6 Dhyana: 33
   3.2.7 Relaxation: 33
   3.2.8 Appliance of Yoga Therapy : 34

4. REVIEW OF LITERATURE	35
5. MATERIALS AND METHODS	44
5.1.1 Place of the study	44
5.1.2 Selection of sample	44
5.1.3 Study design:	44
☐ Inclusion criteria	44
☐ Exclusion criteria	44
5.1.5 Ethical clearance	45
5.1.6 Consent:	45
5.1.7 Case history recording:	45
5.1.8 Medical assessment:	45
5.1.9 Collection of blood sample:	45
5.1.10 Parameters:	45
5.2 Hypothesis:	46
5.3 Yoga therapy:	46
5.3.1 Life Style:	47
5.3.2 Asana :	47
5.3.3 Method of practice of Asana :	48
5.3.4 Pranayama:	48
5.3.5 Dhyana :	49
5.3.6 Relaxation :	49
5.4 Statistical Analysis:	49
6 . RESULTS	51
6.1.1 Demographic Characteristics of the subjects chosen for the study:	51
6.1.2 Comparison of pre and post of experimental group subjects:	52
6.1.3 Comparison of pre and post of Control group subjects:	52
6.1.4 Comparison of pre and post test of experimental group of Menorrhagic subjects:	53
6.1.5 Comparison of pre and post test of control group of Menorrhagic subjects :	53
6.1.6 Comparison of experimental and control group: Two sample test.	54
6.1.7 Comparison of pre and post test of experimental group of Oligomenorrhea subjects :	54

- 6.1.8 Comparison of pre and post test of control group of Oligomenorrhea subjects : 55
- 6.1.9 Comparison of experimental and control group: Two sample test. 55
- 6. 12 Comparison of Experimental and Control group 56
- 6. 13 Distribution of Estrogen, LH & Hb in Menorrhagic subjects 57
- 6.14 Distribution of Estrogen, LH & Hb in Oligomenorrhoea subjects 58
- 6.15 Comparision of experimental and control group: Menorrhagia 59
- 6.16 Comparision of experimental and control group: Oligomenorrhoea 60
- 6.10 Summary of effect of yoga on quality of life 60
- 6.11 Summary of test results-Quality of life 61
- 6.17 Graphical representation of quality of life 62
- 6.2. Discussion: 64
- 6.2.1 Estrogen hormone: 64
- 6.2.2 Luteinising Hormone: 65
- 6.2.3 Haemoglobin: 65
- 6.2.4 Assessment of Quality of life: 66
- 6.2.5 Effect of Yoga Therapy on Anaemic condition of Subjects: 66
- 6.2.6 Impact of Yoga Therapy in reducing symptoms of menstrual disorder: 67
- **7. CONCLUSION** 69
- 7.1 Conclusion: 69
- 7.2 Limitations of the study: 69
- 7.3 Suggestion for the future research 69
- **Bibliography** 80

1. INTRODUCTION

1.1 Yoga:

Yoga is a way of life. It is the traditional and cultural science of India. Its aim is to achieve Samadhi, higher state of self-realisation. The Vedas, Upanishads, and Puranas provide undeniable evidence of yoga and yogic methods. Maharsi Patanjali is attributed with describing and structuring yoga in a systematic and comprehensive manner through his Yoga sutras. He interpreted yoga as the process of योगश्चित्तवृत्तिनिरोधः (Vivekananda, 2011). According to him, योगाङ्गऽनुष्ठानादशुद्धिक्षयेज्ञानदीप्तिराविवेकख्यातेः (Vivekananda, 2011), the practise of various limbs of yoga mitigates impurities and increases radiant knowledge until discrimination. The life of a living being is complicated, and it is full of joy, sorrow, attachment, and ignorance. So, yoga is a way to be free of dualities in order to attain a state of knowledge, the correct direction for locating the state of samadhi, which is the most essential state in which one can be free of life, death, old age, illness, etc.

One of the aims of yoga is to encourage positive hygiene and health (Kuvalyananda)व्याधिस्त्यानसंशयप्रमादालस्याविरतिभ्रान्तिदर्शनालब्धभूमिकत्वानवस्थितत्वानिचित्तविक्षेपास्तेऽन्तरायाः means, physical and mental disease are the main obstructing distractions in life. Classical Yoga texts, such as Hathapradipika, emphasise the health benefits of Yoga practise and the role of health in achieving the goal of Yoga. Positive health entails more than just the absence of disease; it often involves a jubilant and energising sense of well-being, as well as a degree of general resistance and the ability to cultivate energy against particular offending agents. The practise of yoga limbs can provide a number of health benefits. Yoga therapy, which is the application of effective yogic techniques for various health issues, is offered to the individual to achieve physical and mental health. Yoga is a useful tool in diagnosing many problems in clinical medicine (K, 1998). Modern lifestyle has had an impact in the form of stress, which contributes to psychosomatic disorders. Despite the fact that yoga is not intended for therapy, it has proven to be a very successful treatment for the majority of psychosomatic disorders.

1.2 Yoga Therapy:

It is the systematic application of curative and preventive aspects of yoga given to the person, after considering the nature and the individual as a whole. Regular Yoga practise aims to alleviate diseases, increase vigour, endurance, and agility, and improves the qualities of positivity and self-control. Various classical texts of yoga like Hathapradipika, Gheranda Samhita, Yoga Rahasya, etc explains the yoga therapy according to the state of doshas of an individual. Tridosa, panchamahabhuta, Dhatu, and Mala must be in a healthy condition to preserve health, as any deficiency in these elements will manifest various diseases and disorders both physically and mentally. Most of the illnesses, according to yoga, have their origins in the mind. The mind has a range of effects on the body. Disturbances in the mind affect the physical body, causing normal body functions to become unbalanced and irregular. Yoga is the only method capable of reaching the deepest level from the gross to the subtle stages of the body and mind.

1.3 Background of the study:

Every individual in the modern era is employed in some function. This fast-paced lifestyle has had a major effect on women's health around the world. Their health has deteriorated as a result of their everyday responsibilities, inconsistent lifestyle, irregular eating habits, and lack of sleep. Many women in the twenty-first century are educated and want to work, but the majority of them struggle to balance work and family life. This has a physical and emotional effect on her. Menstruation, fertility, abortion, pregnancy, sexually transmissible diseases, chronic health conditions like endometriosis and polycystic ovary syndrome, and menopause are all related to particular life stages of women's sexual and reproductive health.

In terms of function, deficiency, and disease, the reproductive system is vital to women's health. Health is characterised as a state of full physical, mental, and social well-being, not just the absence of disease or infirmity, according to the World Health Organization's constitution. This is nowhere as relevant and applicable as in the area of reproductive health. Apart from the absence of illness or infirmity, reproductive health refers to people's ability to reproduce, control their fertility, and engage in and enjoy sexual relationships. Due to disturbances in menstrual and reproductive functions many women suffer for the rest of their lives (Anand, 2018). Menstrual health is mostly neglected priority within the sexual and reproductive health domain (Sharma, 2014). The regularity of a woman's menstrual cycle is influenced by a variety of internal and external factors that affect her mind and body. The menstrual cycle can be absent, excessive, abnormal, or cause irritation and extreme pain due to a number of factors. It is then classified as a menstrual disorder (M.M., 2005).

Various researches have been done in this area to cure these symptoms of menstrual disorder. The aim of this study is to discover an alternative and genuine approach to menstrual disorder via yoga, to assess the effects of yoga on menstrual disorder symptoms and to enhance the quality of life of menstrual disorder patients, as well as to standardise yogic practises to prevent, handle, and cure menstrual disorder.

1.4 Relevance of the study:

Since health is the most important aspect of life, and if one does not have good health, he would be unable to experience life's success and prosperity (G, Yoga Therapy in Menstrual Disorders, 2017).The present study discovers the techniques in yoga therapy and will provide standard, analytical and heuristic evidence on the effect of yoga therapy on hormonal levels in subjects with menstrual disorder. Asanas help in improving the functioning of endocrine glands (K, 1998). Yoga also corrects the disorder and prevents the body from malfunctioning. It provides relaxation to body by working through the special senses (K, 1998). This helps also in acquiring knowledge about how yoga therapy can improve the quality of life. Here one can able to see the preventive and curative aspect of yoga therapy which helps in building healthy society.

1.5 Objectives of the study:

- To assess the effect of yoga therapy on hormone levels like estrogen and Luteinizing hormone in subjects with menstrual disorder.
- To analyse the outcome of yoga in improving haemoglobin level.

- To evaluate the quality of life in subjects with menstrual disorder.

1.6 Hypothesis:

It will be hypothesized, as a result of yoga practice.

• There will be normalisation of hormonal levels in the subjects.

• There will be I mprovement in the Haemoglobin level.

• There will be reduction in the symptoms of menstrual disorder.

4. REVIEW OF LITERATURE

A literature review includes current knowledge, as well as important findings and philosophical contributions to a subject. Yoga knowledge can be found in abundance in classical texts. The ultimate aim of yoga is to achieve samadhi, which includes good health. Yoga was described by Maharshi Patanjali as योगश्चित्तवृत्तिनिरोधः (Vivekananda, 2011). The Patanjala Yoga Sutra bestows a range of therapeutic benefits. Yoga's curative, preventive, and promotional elements all relate to human health. The cause of illness, according to Patanjali, is mental distraction. There are examples in classical yoga texts about how to conquer disturbances, which are the source of most diseases. The key reasons for diagnosing and treating ancient methods that are explained in classical texts are pancakosa theory, sadvimsati tattva theory, and tridosa. According to Nathamuni's Yoga Rahasya, women have a special right to practise yoga when compared to men (Krishnamacharya, 2003). It is also claimed that when a woman's body is taken over by disease, it fails to serve its function i.e conception (Krishnamacharya, 2003). As a result, some essential angas of yoga that keep the body safe must be practised by women with some discipline for the family's safety. As a result, every woman on the planet has a special right to practise yoga. Yoga has been the topic of various studies, but the idea of yoga for women health is still isolated.

5. A study by Shabnam Omidvar explained the South Indian unmarried women's menstrual patterns. The incidence of irregular menstruation is high among young females, and menstrual pain has an effect on their ability to function. During menstruation, the majority of the participants had painful menstruation, and three-quarters of them had mild to moderate pain. Adult females complained of severe menstrual pain. Tiredness (47.9%) and back pain were the most common symptoms during menstruation (38.3%). According to the findings of this research, adolescent females have a high prevalence of menstrual irregularities and dysmenorrhea throughout menstruation (Omidvar, Menstrual pattern among unmarried women from south India, 2011).

6. Rani K evaluated A randomised controlled trial looked at the effects of Yoga Nidra on patients with menstrual disturbances' psychological well-being. A total of 150 female participants were recruited for this study, and they were divided into two groups of 75 each. All of the subjects (Cases and controls) were assessed for psychological general well-being (tool) for the first time at the start (baseline) and then again after six months. Anxiety decreased significantly (P= 0.003) and depression decreased significantly (P = 0.01) in the Yoga community after the yoga session. After six months of Yoga therapy (Yoga Nidra), positive wellbeing and general health improved significantly (P0.02), and vitality improved significantly (P0.01) in the Yoga community relative to the control group. Yoga Nidra (yogic relaxation therapy) was found to be successful in treating psychological issues in patients with menstrual disorders. Anxiety and depression levels in yoga groups were substantially lower. After six months of yoga therapy, there has been a noticeable increase in overall fitness, vitality, and wellness (Yoga Nidra) (Rani K. , Impact of Yoga Nidra on psychological general wellbeing in patients with menstrual irregularities: A randomized controlled tria, 2011).
7. Khushbhu Rani conducted Six-month trial of Yoga Nidra in menstrual disorder patients: Effects on somatoform symptoms. They selected 150 female patients randomly and divided into two groups of 75 in each, in which one group had Yoga Nidra intervention and medication and the other was without Yoga Nidra intervention only medication. The thesis made use of a technique called a schedule for clinical evaluation of neuropsychiatry. After 6 months of Yoga Nidra therapy, there was a substantial increase in pain symptoms (P=0.006), gastrointestinal symptoms (P= 0.04), cardiovascular symptoms (P=0.02), and urogenital symptoms (P= 0.005) in the Intervention group compared to the control group. Yoga Nidra is an effective treatment for both recent and long-term psychological disturbances, especially anxiety and depression in women with menstrual disorders. According to the findings, a programme focused on yogic intervention can reduce somatoform symptoms in patients with menstrual disorder (Yoga Nidra) (Rani K. , Six-month trial of

Yoga Nidra in menstrual disorder patients: Effects on somatoform symptoms, 2011).

8. In a study by Nidhi R et al, on adolescents with PCOS, a 12-week holistic yoga programme is substantially more effective than a physical exercise programme in reducing anxiety symptoms. Whitney-Mann The U test was used to compare the scores between the two groups, and it revealed that the differences in state anxiety after the intervention were not statistically significant (P=0.243), while the yoga community (-12.27) saw a significant decrease in exercise group.The improvements in trait anxiety were substantially different between the two groups after 12 weeks of intervention and 5 days of detraining, with the yoga community (−14.97) experiencing a greater reduction than the exercise group (−7.42). The study ended with the suggestion that yoga be used as a complementary treatment for adolescents with PCOS, as it may help to slow the progression of the condition (Nidhi, 2012).

9. A study by M. Rani (2013), Yoga Nidra has been shown to improve hormone profiles in patients with menstrual disturbances. The yogic intervention, also known as yoga nidra, was offered for six months at a rate of 40 minutes per day, five days a week. Both groups' hormonal profiles were assessed at baseline and six months later. Thyroid-stimulating hormone (p0.002), follicle-stimulating hormone (p0.02), luteinizing hormone (p0.001), and prolactin (p0.02) were significantly lower in the intervention group than in the control group in patients with hormone imbalances such as Dysmenorrhoea, Oligomenorrhoea, Menorrhagia, Metrorrhagia, and Hypomenorrhoea (Rani M. , 2013).

10. Usha Nag et al studied Yoga's effectiveness as an alternative treatment for primary dysmenorrhoea and stress were investigated. A total of 113 women with primary dysmenorrhoea and stress were randomly assigned to the research and control groups for this study. For three months, study groups were offered a regular 60-minute yoga session. In the study population, there

was a substantial reduction in pain (p0.0001) after yoga intervention. When compared to the control group, 88 percent of the study group recorded total pain relief and 12 percent reported moderate pain, 82 percent of the study group reported complete stress relief, absenteeism declined to 10%, and physical activity improved. The study concluded that yogic exercises reduced stress and pain associated with dysmenorrhoea, indicating the advantages of yoga in primary dysmenorrhoea. Yoga is beneficial to menstrual health when practised by college students (Nag, 2013).

11. Ramanath et al, tested effect of yoga on anaemic patients in a randomised control trial. For 90 days, 40 subjects were chosen at random and given trikona and its variations, Sarvanga, Surya namaskara, and Yoga mudra. The heart rate, blood pressure, and haemoglobin level of nearly 87.5 percent of the subjects improved. All anaemic patients showed various beneficial results such as pulse rate, blood pressure, and haemoglobin after practising dhyan, asanas, and pranayam for three months (Ramanath, 2013).

12. Ekta et al studied the role of yoga in primary dysmenorrhea, as well as the effects of various asanas on the body. Asanas are said to increase flexibility, relax the body, and balance the sympathetic and parasympathetic nervous systems. Diaphragmatic breathing is aided by relaxation and meditation, which relieves physical and emotional stresses. They came to the conclusion that yoga is a safe therapy. It calms the nervous system and controls the endocrine system. Yoga practise lowers the levels of prostaglandins and inflammatory mediators, which are responsible for pain. It brings body and mind into balance (Ekta, 2014).

13. In a study by Vungarala Satyanand , Yogasanas were tested for their effectiveness in the treatment of menstrual pain. For three months, a case group of 50 participants attended a 45-minute yoga session, and they saw positive results in the treatment of irregular menstruation and the relief of menstrual discomfort. For both classes, a visual analogue scale (VAS) was used to assess pain intensity. Yoga and relaxation exercises were found to be helpful in managing irregular menstruation and reducing discomfort during

menstruation because Yogasana helps to balance both the body and mind. Yoga breathing exercises aided in the improvement of fitness as well as the prevention and treatment of diseases. The findings of this study indicate that in the case community, there was a highly significant increase in positive well-being and vitality (Satyanand, 2014).

14. N Tejwani, in their study titled "Effect of Yoga on Menstrual Disorder," 50 women with menstrual disorders were recruited and given daily yoga classes for six months. A questionnaire was used as a method before and after the research to determine the impact of yoga. When compared to the remaining 12 abnormal subjects, 38 of the 50 subjects continued yoga exercise and showed positive and substantial symptomatic relief. Women with dysmenorrhoea saw a noticeable change in 88 percent of cases. 60 percent of women with menorrhagia saw a decrease in the volume and frequency of their bleeding. Women suffering from PMS reaped the most benefits (96.6 %). Teenagers with irregular menstrual cycles were found to profit in 94 percent of cases. They came to the conclusion that every woman experiences menstrual disturbances at some point in her life, and that gynaecological issues can be handled and avoided by practising yoga (asana, pranayam, relaxation, and concentration techniques) (Tejwani, 2015).

15. Shanti P' s a single case report, six months of yoga practise for 15- 30 minutes twice a day enabled the case's menstrual cycle to be more normal. The case stated that she only experienced moderate pain on the first day of menstruation, which was extreme prior to beginning yoga. It also assisted in the reduction of body weight from 98 to 95 kilogrammes. Yoga's efficacy and stress reduction were noted by the participants. They came to the conclusion that a series of asanas, pranayama, and yoga nidra assisted the subject in losing weight and reducing menstrual pain. If yoga is practised daily from adolescence onwards, one would undoubtedly feel more at ease during menstruation, pregnancy, the postpartum period, and the menopausal period (P, 2015).

16. Neena Sharma & Ritu Gupta, studied yoga's effectiveness in anaemic patients In both men and women, the study found a substantial rise in haemoglobin (p 0.0001) and RBC (p 0.0001). Both men (p 0.0001) and women (p 0.0001) had substantially lower WBC counts. After two months of yoga practice, the mean value of platelet count increased in both men and women, but the difference was statistically insignificant in men (p = 0.3798) and women (p = 0.3479). After obtaining this finding, they concluded that yoga is a low-cost and low-cost discipline that can be used as a drug-free therapy for improving anaemic patients' haematological parameters. Yoga's anti-stress and antioxidant properties increase blood supply and the overall function of the circulatory system (Neena Sharma, 2016) .

17. Govardhan Reddy, in his article entitled Asanas help to improve the activity of the endocrine glands, according to Yoga Therapy in Menstrual Disorders. It also encourages body stability so that muscles do not get damaged. Asana practise helps to stretch the pelvic muscles on a regular basis. Breathing exercises boost lung capacity while also relaxing the entire body by reducing stress and anxiety. Daily Yoga practise was found to be helpful in the prevention and treatment of menstrual disorders, as well as promoting general health, relaxation, and stress reduction. It also helps to enhance psychological responses during the menstrual cycle (G, Yoga Therapy in Menstrual Disorders, 2017).

18. Oates J, reviewed 15 studies described in 18 papers in which range of yoga therapies, which included a combination of asana, pranayam, and other yogic relaxation or meditation strategies, were found to alleviate menstrual pain symptoms. All of the included studies indicated some improvement in their outcome measures, indicating that a yoga intervention decreased menstrual pain symptoms; however, the heterogeneity and severity of the interventions and outcome measures restricted the generalizability and applicability of the results in practise settings. They concluded that further study on yoga and menstrual disorders is inevitable, but that accuracy of methodology and

efficiency must be prioritised so that results can be replicated outside of clinical trials (Oates, 2017).

19. A study by Nazish Rafique, studied the prevalence of menstrual problems and their relationship to psychological stress in young female students studying health sciences was studied, and it was discovered that menstrual problems are more common as a result of academic stress. They also noted that a variety of factors, such as age, dietary habits, family background, ethnicity, and physical activity, can influence menstrual pattern. Stress, on the other hand, may be a significant contributor to menstrual irregularities. Irregular menstruation (27%) was the most common concern, followed by amenorrhoea (9.2%), menorrhagia (3.4%), and dysmenorrhoea (3.4%). (89.7%). According to the findings, stress-related menstrual problems are common in young girls. Premenstrual symptom, amenorrhea, dysmenorrhea, and psychological stress were all found to be strongly linked in this study (N, 2018).

20. Shabnam Omidvar et al studied the pattern of Indian teenage girls in a South Indian urban area was studied. 536 healthy menstruating females aged 10 to 19 years were recruited for this study, and they were given To collect relevant data, standardised self-reporting questionnaires were used. Chi-square or Fisher's exact tests were used to evaluate categorical results. The results revealed that 73.1 percent of people had cycles that lasted 21–35 days. More than half of them said their menstrual blood flow lasted 5–6 days, and 12% said it lasted more than 7 days. Thirty percent said they had lost a lot of blood. Dymenorrhoea affected 66.8% of the women (Omidvar, 2018).

21. In a study by Sonal Kulshrestha conducted a course of ten months, 320 adolescent schoolgirls aged 14-17 years participated in a cross-sectional descriptive study to determine the overall prevalence of menstrual disorders. A predesigned pretested standardised questionnaire cum interview schedule was used to collect data on age at menarche, menstrual cycle interval, menstrual flow duration, and period pain. To determine the level of physical activity The PAQ-A (physical activity questionnaire scale) was used. The total incidence of menstrual disorders was 76.9%, with dysmenorrhoea accounting for 46.3

percent, amenorrhoea 21.3 percent, oligomenorrhoea 12.8 percent, polymenorrhoea 22.2 percent, menorrhagia 15.9%, and hypomenorrhoea 15%.Physical activity must be recognised as a major and relevant risk factor when defining various forms of menstrual disorders, according to the findings (Kulshrestha, 2019).

22. Monika Singh et al, studied menstrual trends and issues in 210 Delhi teenage school girls in relation to body mass index. Weight, personal data, age of menarche in years, regularity, and anthropometric examination were all reported using a standardised weighing scale. A questionnaire was used to gather data on menstruation-related issues such as complications during the menstrual cycle. SPSS 17.0 was used to analyse the data. Out of 210 adolescent girls, 114 (54.3%) had a BMI of 18.5 or less, indicating that more than half of the girls were malnourished. Only 13 adolescent girls (6.2 percent) were overweight. Symptoms and problems associated with menstrual cycles were more common in adolescent girls with a BMI of 18.5 or less.The disparity between the two groups was statistically important. It was discovered that teenage girls suffer from dysmenorrhoea, which has an effect on their lives and outdoor activities. BMI is extremely important for menstrual cycle regularity. As a result, adolescent girls must be provided with a safe and balanced diet in order to maintain a regular BMI and control their menstrual cycles (Singh, 2019).

23. Enu Anand surveyed about Neglect of Menstrual Disorders in Reproductive Health Care in India: A Population-Based Survey and is about the prevalence of menstrual health problems and their association with various socio-economic, demographic, and reproductive health factors using a population-based survey. Here it is clear that Menstrual health problems are a largely neglected priority within the sexual and reproductive health domain in most low-income countries. Report showed that Pain during menstruation (5.6%) and irregular menstrual cycles (4.3%) were most common (Anand, 2018).

24. Shraddha Prabhu in their study on Effect Of Yogasanas On Menstrual Cramps highlighted the importance of performing yogasanas and as a non-

pharmacological form of treatment. The VMSS and Moo's MDQ questionnaires showed a substantial difference (P 0.05), but the PSS score (P 0.641) did not vary significantly in either community. Both yogasanas and core exercises will help with menstrual pain, according to the findings. These are inexpensive and can be achieved at home to increase one's quality of life and menstrual well-being. The VMSS and Moo's MDQ questionnaires showed a substantial difference (P 0.05), but the PSS score (P 0.641) did not vary significantly in either community. Both yogasanas and core exercises will help with menstrual pain, according to the findings. These are inexpensive and can be achieved at home to increase one's quality of life and menstrual well-being. (Prabhu, 2019)

2. MENSTRUAL DISORDER

2.1 Overview of menstrual disorder:

Puberty and reproductive functions of female occurs by hormonal changes which are regulated by the female reproductive system. Coalescing of hormonal signal from the hypothalamus, pituitary and ovary emanate in repetitive series of follicle development, ovulation and formation of the endometrial lining of the uterus for implantation. This complex and highly synchronised pattern of events that exhibit as menstruation check that only one oocyte is ovulated in one cycle and if the fertilization does not occur the process of endometrial shedding takes place (Edmonds, 2007).

2.2 Menstruation:

Menstruation is the viewable manifestation of periodic uterine bleeding due to shedding of the endometrium (Dutta, Textbook Of Gynecology, 2013). Hypothalamus-pituitary-ovarian function regulates the periodicity of the menstruation and loss of blood depends on the condition of the uterus (Howkins, 2000).It is the monthly course of changes in the ovaries and endometrium commencing with the anticipation of an egg for fertilisation. Ovulation occurs when the follicles of prepared egg in the ovary rupture, it is liberated for fertilization. This cycle ends with the shedding of part of endometrium and is called menstruation, unless pregnancy occurs. Duration of this cycle is about three to five days and 50ml to 200ml blood loss is estimated (Howkins, 2000).

2.3 Importance of menstruation:

The woman body prepares for pregnancy every month and it is the lining of the uterus that gets thicker as spadework for regular menstruation. This shows that there is hormonal balance within the body. Fertilization of egg occurs in the lining of the uterus and if egg is not fertilised, uterine lining starts to breakdown and is expelled through vagina. Menstruation is the way of releasing the uterine tissue that it no longer needs. If menstrual cycle is not normal, then it is considered as disorder of menstruation, which disrupts her daily life. It can also affect her ability to conceive.

All around the world major problem faced by women are menstrual disorders and generally less concern is paid to understanding women's menstrual complaints Menstrual irregularities influence on the daily life of the females. High risk of depression can be seen along with menstrual irregularity and heavy menstrual flow (BL, 2004).

2.4 Menstrual Disorders:

It is an abnormal condition in menstrual cycle which affects the quality of life of the women and is the signal of serious underlying problems. Reciprocity action between hypothalamus, pituitary, ovary and uterus is the leads to proper monthly menstruation. Disordered menstruation occurs when there disturbance at any point of axis (Edmonds, 2007). Various factors have impact on the pattern of menstruation. Due to menstrual disturbances, physical and psychological repercussions are faced by majority of girls in student category which impose to absenteeism and also can cause problems in their families.

2.5 Prevalence of menstrual disorder:

In a study done in Aligarh city in India, the overall prevalence of menstrual disorders was reported by 76.9%. The most common menstrual disorder was PMS 71.3%. Dysmenorrhoea was 46.3%, amenorrhoea 21.3%, oligomenorrhea 12.8%, polymenorrhea 22.2%, menorrhagia 15.9% and hypomenorrhea 15% (SonalKulshrestha, 2019) .It was foundthe rate of lower abdominal pain or vaginal discharge with fever was 16%, and menstrual bleeding disorders or pain 15% (JC, 1997).

2.6 Aetiology of menstrual disorder:

Menstrual disorders can have variety of causes such as hormonal imbalance, prolonged strenuous exercise program, eating disorders, hypothalamic dysfunction, tumours in pituitary gland, ovary or adrenal gland, long-term use of drugs like steroidal oral contraceptives (Sembulingam, Essentials of medical physiology, 2016). Other causes such as uterine fibroids, bleeding disorders, cancer, sexually transmitted infections, polycystic ovary syndrome- cysts on the ovaries, genetics may also cause disorder of menstruation.

- ➢ Hormonal imbalance: Lower levels of estrogen hormone are usually associated with Amenorrhea (Jameson, 2010). Imbalance of thyroid hormone can also cause irregularity in menstruation.
- ➢ Uterine fibroids: Irregular bleeding and pelvic pain occur due to abnormal growth in the walls of the uterus called fibroids. Estrogen and progesterone play a role in the growth of fibroids.

2.7 Types of menstrual disorder:

1. Ammenorrhoea:

   Deprivation or abnormal cessation of the menses is called ammenorrhoea (Philadelphia, 2000). Natural causes for amenorrhoea are pregnancy, breast feeding and menopause. Factors like Lifestyle, excessive exercise, medication use, hormone imbalances and structural issues and stress can cause amenorrhoea. Infertility can occur due to amenorrhea and when amenorrhoea is caused by low level of estrogen there is higher possibility of osteoporosis.

2. Oligomenorrhoea:

   It is the decreased frequency of menstrual bleeding (Sembulingam, 2016). Menstrual periods at intervals of more than 35 days or irregular periods with unpredictable flow are the symptoms. Adolescent girls are more vulnerable to oligomenorrhoea.

3. Hypomenorrhea:

   Menstrual bleeding is decreased. The menstruation often lasts less than two days, or it is less than 80ml. Lower body fat, nervousness or stress, hormonal imbalance, premature ovarian failure etc may the aetiological factors for hypomenorrhea.

4. Menorrhagia:

   Abnormally heavy or prolonged bleeding. Menorrhagia may occur due to dysfunction in the ovaries, uterine fibroids, and hormone imbalance. One may have to use more than one sanitary pad every hour for several consecutive hours. Blood clots can be seen and bleeding can last for more than a week that may result in anaemia and fatigue that restrict daily activities of the person.

5. Polymenorrhea:

    Increased frequency of menstruation (Sembulingam, 2016). The menstrual cycle is shorter than 21 days. The causes for polymenorrhea may be stress, hormonal fluctuations etc.

6. Metrorrhagia:

    Uterine bleeding in between menstruations (Sembulingam, 2016) . It is a sign of an underlying disorder, and it may lead to anaemia.

7. Painful menstruation/ dysmenorrhea:

    This means painful menstruation (Dutta, 2013). Pelvic congestion or increased Vascularity in the pelvic organs results in dysmenorrheoa (Dutta, 2013). Just before and during menstrual period hindering pains in the lower abdomen are experienced. This pain radiate to the lower back and thighs. Nausea, vomiting, diarrhea or constipation, headache, dizziness, hypersensitivity to sound, light and certain smell are the symptoms which can be seen along with menstrual pain.

    - Primary dysmenorrhea: The primary dysmenorrhea is one where there is no identifiable pelvic pathology. Causes for this primary dysmenorrhea may be tension and anxiety during adolescence and abnormal anatomical and functional aspect of myometrium (Dutta, 2013).
    - Secondary dysmenorrhea: It's a form of pain that happens when there's a problem with the pelvis. Secondary dysmenorrhoea may be caused by a number of factors, including chronic pelvic infection, pelvic endometriosis, pelvic adhesions, adenomyosis, uterine fibroid, endometrial polyp, and pelvic congestion (Dutta, 2013).

8. Pre Menstrual Disorder (PMS):

    Is a psychoneuroendocrine condition that occurs just before menstruation. The cause of PMS is unclear. Anxiety, depression, mood swings, irritability, headache, insomnia, fatigue, , are some of the symptoms.

2.8 Role of hormones:

- Estrogen: It is primarily secreted by ovarian follicles and in small amounts by the corpus luteum of the ovaries. It produces a lot of secretion at the end of the follicular process, just before ovulation. It is present in three forms in plasma. β-estradiol, Estrone, Estriol. The level of estrogen in plasma varies during different phases of menstrual cycle (Sembulingam, 2016).

    Functions of estrogen: Estrogen's primary role is to promote cellular proliferation and tissue growth, especially in the sexual organs. It enhances cilia function and increases blood flow to the endometrium, allowing the ovum to pass more easily. Estrogen is responsible for the production of secondary sexual features such as hairs in the pubic region and the axilla. It enhances bone development during puberty. Osteoporosis is caused by a loss of oestrogen secretion in old age or during menopause (Sembulingam, 2016).

    Regulation of Estrogen secretion: Anterior pituitary releases follicle stimulating hormone by the stimulation of gonadotropin- releasing hormone. FSH regulates the secretion of estrogen (Sembulingam, 2016).

- Luteinising hormone: It is a glycoprotein that is needed for ovulation to occur. Also with a significant amount of FSH, ovulation does not occur without LH. Ovulatory surge for LH, also known as luteal surge, is the need for excessive LH secretion for ovulation. Due to the positive feedback effect of oestrogen on GnRH, a significant amount of LH is secreted prior to ovulation (Sembulingam, 2016).

    Functions of LH: It causes maturation of vesicular follicle into graafian follicle along with follicle-stimulating hormone. It is responsible for ovulation and formation of corpus luteum (Sembulingam, 2016).

- Haemoglobin:

    The iron-containing colouring matter of red blood cells is called haemoglobin. Haemoglobin's main function is to transport respiratory gases, such as oxygen from the lungs to the tissues and carbon dioxide from the tissues to the lungs. Haemoglobin levels in females should be between 12.1 and 15.1 g/dL. (Sembulingam, 2016). Hemoglobin deficiency may be caused by a reduction in the number of haemoglobin molecules in the blood, as in anaemia, or by a decrease in each molecule's ability to bind oxygen at the same partial pressure of oxygen, as in hypoxia. The loss of red blood cells during menorrhagia or excessive blood loss during menstruation may cause anaemia. Haemoglobin counts the number of red blood cells in the body. The body tries to compensate for the missing red blood cells by using iron reserves to produce more haemoglobin, which can then hold oxygen on red blood cells, resulting in iron deficiency anaemia. Menorrhagia can lower iron levels to the point that iron deficiency anaemia is a possibility.

3. YOGIC MANAGEMENT OF MENSTRUAL DISORDER:

3.1 Rajodarsana/ Menstruation

मासि मासि रजः स्त्रीणां रसजं स्रवति व्यहम् ।
वत्सराद्द्वादशादूर्ध्वं याति पञ्चाशतः क्षयम् ॥

After the age of twelve years, rajas (menstrual blood), which is the result of rasa (the first dhatu), flows out of the body for three days per month, and by the age of fifty years, it has diminished (Murthy, Vagbhata's Astanga Hrdayam, 1991).

वातादिकुष्णपग्रन्थिपूयक्षीणमलाह्वयम् ।
बीजासमर्थं रेतोऽष्टम् स्वलिङ्गैर्दोषजं वदेत् ॥
रक्तेन कुणपं, श्लेष्मवाताभ्यां ग्रन्थिसन्निभम् ।
पूयाभं रक्तपित्ताभ्यां, क्षीणं मारुतपित्ततः ॥
कृच्छ्राण्येतान्यसाध्यं तु त्रिदोषं मूत्रविट्प्रभम् ।

Retas (semen) and asra (menstrual blood), also known as vitiated by vata, vitiated by pitta, vitiated by kapha, retas (semen), retas (semen), retas (semen), retas (semen), retas (semen), retas (semen), reta (masses, pellets). That resembles pus, that has reduced in quantity, and that smells like waste (mutra-urine) and purisa (feces)- are unable to develop the embryo (Murthy, 1991).

Types of yoni roga:

- Vataja yoni roga :

मिथ्याचारेण ताः स्त्रीणां प्रदुष्टेनार्तवेन च।
जायन्ते बीजदोषाच्च दैवाच्च शृणु ताः पृथक्॥

Charaka samhita chikitsasana 30th - 8

Uterine ailments are caused by mitachara (wrong regime), pradusta arthava (menstrual morbidities), beeja dosha(defective genes, ovum), daiva or karma (https://niimh.nic.in/ebooks/ecaraka/).

वातलाहारचेष्टाया वातलायाः समीरणः।
विवृद्धो योनिमाश्रित्य योनेस्तोदं सवेदनम्।।
स्तम्भं पिपीलिकासृप्तिमिव कर्कशतां तथा।
करोति सुप्तिमायासं वातजांश्चापरान् गदान्।।
सा स्यात् सशब्दरुक्फेनतनुरूक्षार्तवाऽनिलात्।

Charaka samhita chikitsasana 30th – 9-10

The aggravated vata in women's body effects on her reproductive organs to produce some symptoms such as stambha (stiffness or numbness), pipilika (a sensation as if ants are crawling), supti (numbness in reproductive organs), untimely menstrual bleeding which is phena (frothy), tanu (thin), ruksha (dry) and associated with sound and pain (https://niimh.nic.in/ebooks/ecaraka/).

- Pittaja Yoni roga:

व्यापत्कटुम्लवणक्षाराद्यैः पित्तजा भवेत्।।
दाहपाकज्वरोष्णार्ता नीलपीतासितार्तवा।
भृशोष्णकुणपस्रावा योनिः स्यात्पित्तदूषिता।।

Charaka samhita chikitsasana 30th – 11-12

The aggravated pitta in women's body effects on her reproductive organs to produce some symptoms such as daha (burning sensation), paka (suppuration), jwara (fever), usna(heat), menstrual bleeding becomes nila, pita, sita (blue, yellow, black) in color, bhrsha (large quantity), kunapa (smells like a dead body) (https://niimh.nic.in/ebooks/ecaraka/).

- Kaphaja Yoni roga:

कफोऽभिष्यन्दिभिर्वृद्धो योनिं चेद्दूषयेत् स्त्रियाः।
स कुर्यात् पिच्छिलां शीतां कण्डुग्रस्ताल्पवेदनाम्।।
पाण्डुवर्णां तथा पाण्डुपिच्छिलार्तववाहिनीम्।

Charaka samhita chikitsasana 30th – 13

The aggravated pitta in women's body effects on her reproductive organs to produce some symptoms such as picchilam (sliminess), shitam (cold), kandu (itching), vedanam (mild pain), pandu varna(pale colored genital organ), pandu picchila arthava vahinim (pale and slimy menstrual discharge) (https://niimh.nic.in/ebooks/ecaraka/).

- Arajaska/ Amenorrhea:

योनिगर्भाशयस्थं चेत् पित्तं सन्दूषयेदसृक्।
साऽरजस्का मता काश्यैवैवर्ण्यजननी भृशम्।।

Charaka samhita chikitsasana 30th – 17

When pitta is located in the uterus, then there will no menstruation i.e arajaska or amenorrhea(7).

- Pradara/ Asrdagara or menorrhagia:

यः पूर्वमुक्तः प्रदरः शृणु हेत्वादिभिस्तु तम्।।
याऽत्यर्थं सेवते नारी लवणाम्लगुरूणि च।
कटूंन्यथ विदाहीनि स्निग्धानि पिशितानि च।।
ग्राम्यौदकानि मेद्यानि कृशरां पायसं दधि।
शुक्तमस्तुसुरादीनि भजन्त्याः कुपितोऽनिलः।।
रक्तं प्रमाणमुत्क्रम्य गर्भाशयगताः सिराः।
रजोवहाः समाश्रित्य रक्तमादाय तद्रजः।।
यस्माद्विवर्धयत्याशु रसभावाद्विमानता।
तस्मादसृग्दरं प्राहुरेतत्तन्त्वविशारदाः।।
रजः प्रदीर्यते यस्मात् प्रदरस्तेन स स्मृतः।
सामान्यतः समुद्दिष्टं कारणं लिङ्गमेव च।।
चतुर्विधं व्यासतस्तु वाताद्यैः सन्निपाततः।

Charaka samhita chikitsasana 30th – 204-208

If a woman consume excess of saline, sour, pungent, unctuous food, krsara(a preparation of rice & pulses), payasa (a preparation of milk & ghee), sura(a type of alcohol), vata in her body gets aggravated. This aggravated vayu increases the quantity of menstrual blood. This is called Pradara/ Asrdagara or menorrhagia. There are four types of pradara, namely vatika pradara, paittika pradara, kaphaja pradara and sannipatika pradara (https://niimh.nic.in/ebooks/ecaraka/).

According to Nathamuni's *Yoga Rahasya,*

अधिकारो विशेषेण स्त्रीणां पुंभ्यो निगद्यते ।
सन्तानतरु विस्तारे स्त्रीशरीरम् हि कारणम्

-Nathamunis Yoga Rahasya – 1-14

Women have a special right to practise yoga as opposed to men. This is because she is the one who maintains the lineage's continuity (Krishnamacharya, 2003).

It is also said,

यथा तद्वत् रुजाक्रान्तं स्त्रीशरीरं निरर्थकम् ।
तस्मात् लोके स्त्रियः सर्वाः विशेषेणाधिकारिणः

- NathamunisYoga Rahasya– 1-16

Women have a special right to practise yoga and when a woman's body is taken over by illness, she loses her ability to conceive (Krishnamacharya, 2003). It is beneficial to both men and women. As the responsibilities of women are greater than men, there is more requirement of yoga. Menstrual disorders may be explained according to the principles of yoga therapy as follows:

3.1.1 Tridosha theory:

The tridoshas in human body according to tridosha theory are vata, pitta and kapha.Health is a state where there is balanced condition of these doshas and its imbalance is considered as diseased or being ill. They unitedly sustain the body.Discrepancy of vata in the body leads to menstrual disorders. In the lower part of the body i.e below the pelvic region, resides the apana vayu and its malfunction causes vata to become vitiated.The Apana vayu is responsible for the proper functioning of the reproductive system. Vitiation of kapha and pitta resulting in foul smelling, increased quantity, clots in menstrual flow. Increased kapha is a symptom of menorrhagia.Endometrial tissue development is more pronounced as kapha's effect grows higher.Discrepancy in pitta dosha can also influence on heavy bleeding, as pitta is usna(hot) and tikshna (sharp), it brings more fluidity to blood helping in easy flow. It is the cause for swelling and tenderness of breasts before menses. Cholesterol is a precursor for the development of oestrogen and all other steroidal hormones in females. Cholesterol/fat is a kapha whose volume is increased by oestrogen activity, resulting in endometrial hyperplasia and menorrhagia. As the location of vata is below the naval region, it dominates in uterus. Due to the khara(rough) and sheeta (cold & dry) qualities of vata, makes the blood vessels to constrict. Due to its ruksha(dry) guna, body fluids and menstrual flow stop early. Which causes a drop in body fluids, resulting in less nourishment for the uterus' endometrial lining, resulting in a smaller endometrium and less menstrual discharge.

Apana Vata –

अपानोअपानगःश्रोणिवस्तिमेढ्रोरुगोचरः
शुक्रार्तवशकृन्मूत्रगर्भनिष्क्रमणक्रियः॥

- (Astanga hrdaya – 12 दोषभेदयं - 9)

Apana vata is located in the large intestine and moves through the waist, bladder, and genitals. Ejaculation, menstruation, defecation, urination, and childbirth are among the functions it attends to (https://www.planetayurveda.com/ayurveda-ebooks/astanga-hridaya-sutrasthan-handbook.pdf).

अपानकोपतो ये हि व्याधिसंघा उदीरिताः ।
मूलतो ते विनश्यन्ति लोहितस्सरलो भवेत्॥

-NathamunisYoga Rahasya- 1-69

Those diseases caused by a vitiation of the apana vayu are fully eradicated, and the blood becomes clean as well (Krishnamacharya, 2003).

3.1.2 Panchakosha theory:

According to this theory human has an aggregate of five sheaths or koshas called panchakoshas - Annamaya kosha, Pranamaya kosha, Manomaya kosha, Vijnanamaya kosha and Anandamaya kosha. Any abnormalities in Annamaya kosha, Pranamaya kosha, or Manomaya kosha may cause menstrual irregularities. Abnormalities in annamaya kosha is caused by improper consumption of food, both quantity and quality. Unhealthy and unpleasant food consumption leads to vitiation in panchamahabhuta (i.e Increase of prthvi, Ap and Tejas and decrease of vayu and akasa) and in tridosha. The consumption of pathya and mithahara foods aids in the proper functioning of the annamaya kosha. Adapting the yamas, niyamas, kriyas, and asanas as vihara in daily life will help prevent a variety of diseases. Since vitiated doshas (vata, pitta, and kapha) and gunas (rajas and tamas) prevent prana from flowing in the proper direction, the body's rhythm and hormony are disrupted. The stability and steadiness of nadis are lost in this condition resulting in the alteration rhythm of breathing and as a result diseases may be developed. Physiological and psychological homeostasis like pulse rate, heart rate varies and pain/aches develops. By the practice of Pranayama this can be managed through. The eternal cause of thoughts is prana, which can be regulated by the mind. The metabolic processes of digestion, elimination, and even circulation are all hampered by a confused mind. Psychological symptoms related to menstrual disorder are caused by disturbed manas. When there is a disruption in the manomaya kosa, such as stress, tension, fear, anxiety, and so on, it can trigger a corresponding disturbance in the physical level by inducing a hormonal imbalance, resulting in a disrupted menstrual cycle. Similarly when Ap tattva is disrupted, problems with taste and shortness of breath may occur. In karmendriyya level, it is excretory organ that is affected. One may observe the decrease of blood volume in the body. When the tejas tattva s affected, the result can be observed in the eyes. Eyes may be paler in colour in women suffering from anaemia and menorrhagia, and muscle weakness and cramps may develop at the karmendriya stage.Reduced agni/tejas can result in decreased gastric fire, or agnimandya, as well as decreased vision.A disrupted vayu causes numbness/hypoesthesia in the skin at the jnanendriya level, as well as discomfort, numbness, and coldness in the hands and feet at the karmendriya level. When the akasa tattva is upset, reduced auditory functions, balancing and in karmendriya level trouble, headache, voice and coordination difficulties occurs.

सप्तचक्रक्षालनाय वृक्षासनविशेषकान् ।
जननेन्द्रियदार्ढ्याय कोणभेदान् समभ्यसेत् ॥

-Nathamunis Yoga Rahasya-II-20//

Vrksasana is a special asana for cleansing the seven cakras. Different variants of konasana must also be performed to strengthen the reproductive organs (Krishnamacharya, 2003).

बन्धादस्मान्नरस्खलेच्च वीर्यं नृणां कदापि हि ।
स्त्रीणां रजोविशुद्धिश्च जायते न हि संशयः ॥

- Nathamunis Yoga Rahasya - I-80//

A man's virility is vnever lost when he performs this bandha (jalandhara bandha). Women's rajo kosas (reproductive organs) are also cleansed (Krishnamacharya, 2003).

3.1.3 Sadvimshati tattva theory:

This theory explains about evolution of the entire world/universe. Purusha and prakriti unites as a result of disturbance in the equilibrium of triguna (Sattva, rajas, tamas). Hence there occurs manifestation of mahat, ahankara, manas, 5 jnanendriyas, 5 karmendriyas, 5 tanmatras, panchamahabhutas and iswara as 26th entity. As there is correlation between sensor, motor organs, panchamahabhutas and the citta, there is path to find the root of manifestation of disease.

The vayu and akasa tattvas rise during menstruation, while the prthvi, ap, and tajas tattvas fall. Cittavikshepas arise when the balance between the citta, jnanendriya, karmendriya, and mahabhutas is broken, as they are all interconnected. Both tattva levels undergo cyclic effects as a result of these disturbances.

When prthvi tattva is out of control, the function of the corresponding karmendriya, i.e. the Upastha/reproductive organs, is affected. Menstrual behaviours are linked to upastha, and as a result, menstrual disorders such as menorrhagia can occur. Menorrhagia can cause anaemia because when the prthvi tattva is disturbed, it causes problems with the nose at the jnanendriya level and the genital organ at the karmendriya level. Weakness, exhaustion, or a loss of body weight, reduced libido, muscle spasms, and other symptoms are seen at the karmendriya stage.

3.1.4 Principles and approach of yoga therapy:

Yoga therapy gives holistic approach in physical, mental and spiritual levels. In this study, with respect to prevent, cure and manage the menstrual disorder, standardised yoga therapy is used as the tool.

- Physical level: Menstrual irregularities are caused by abnormal metabolic activity and hormone production imbalances. As a consequence, digestion is the most important factor in overcoming this problem. It is the mechanism by which food is transformed into rasa, which is then transformed into Rakta. Menstruation is represented by the quality or guna present in Rakta. By maintaining systematic metabolic and endocrine cycles, yogic practises such as asanas help to preserve the balance of doshas in the body. Asanas help to activate the endocrine system, which helps to balance hormone levels in the bloodstream.

- Mental level: Since the endocrine and nervous systems are intertwined, homeostasis of the HPO axis is required for proper hormone balance in the body. Pranayama is a technique that will help you do this. Pranayama is a method for relaxing the mind and thereby improving mental wellbeing (Krishna, 1998) . Dhyana practise aids in the reduction of mental tension. Cell rejuvenation is aided by relaxation exercises such as savasana. A calm, healthy mind aids in improving the body's ability to function.

- Spiritual level: Women are especially vulnerable to psychological disorders and vulnerability. They are easily affected by psychiatric disturbances, which has an effect on both their physical and mental health. To address this problem, yoga therapy is the only solution, since it encompasses mental, emotional, and social well-being as a holistic spiritual approach.

3.2 Yoga therapy for menstrual disorders:

Yoga is a form of medicine that has been used for hundreds of years as a method for psychological and spiritual evolution and wellbeing (K, 1998). It's a tried-and-true factor whose theories on health and disease have never changed. The relationship between the mind and the body is harmonised by yoga practise. The basic framework for achieving health can only be developed through yoga practise. Yoga not only cures the sickness, but it also changes a person's perspective on health and disease. Yoga therapy is the clinical application of yoga theory to treat different disorders.

Lifestyle modifications, various asanas, pranayamas, bandha, mudra and Dhyana are the different components of yoga therapy.

3.2.1 Lifestyle: Harmony between the body, mind, and soul is the definition of total health. It is attained by a balanced diet, adequate exercise, and a stress-free mind. People suffer from poor posture, body pains, and other ailments as a result of their unhealthy lifestyles (K, 1998). The practise of yamas and niyamas, as well as asana and pranayama, is important for good health. Ahimsa is accomplished by a gentle approach to all. Aparigraha must be practised in order to break the loop of desires. Sauca should be prioritised by the whole family (K, 1998). Spiritual living decreases tension in one's life. As stress levels rise, inner equilibrium is disrupted, and the entire system fails. These can be overcome by leading a safe lifestyle.

3.2.2 Asana: According to Hathapradika, practice of asana brings, steadiness, health and lightness of the body i.e स्थैर्यमारोग्यंचाङ्गलाघवम् (Digambaraji, 1998). It is capable to achieve ततोद्वन्द्वानभिघातः॥ (Vivekananda, 2011) i.e free from dualities. Asana practise aids in the purification of blood and the removal of toxic/impurities from various parts of the body, allowing for adequate blood circulation. This ensures adequate cellular nutrition and balances the nervous system.

Systematic practice with following sequence leads to better result. Each asana has following four components

i. Vinyasa: Sequence of steps in asana.
ii. Svasocchvasa: Breathing pattern to be ensured during performing vinyasa. Synchronisation of vinyasa and svasocchvasa is necessary to deliver better result. Improper breathing leads to negative effect on body and mind.
iii. Sthithi: It is the final position in which the practitioner maintains particular number of svasa.
iv. Drsti: Sthithi of each asana has its own focussing places of eyes like nasagra drsti, angusta drsti, bhrumadhya drsti, antardrsti, bahirdrsti etc.

Asanas performed by this way improves the coordination between mind and body that helps in stimulating and proper functioning of all the body system. This yield in steadiness, health and lightness of the body.

3.2.3 Physiological contributions of asana:

- Swastikasana: It is a fortunate meditative pose that is much easier to execute than other asanas and can be performed by those who are unable to sit in other meditative poses. It's a great asana for pranayama and meditation (K, 1998)[21].
- Vajrasana and Suptavajrasana : It's a excellent meditative asana. It's a very soothing place, ideal for calming the mind and body (S, Yoga and Kriya, 2008). During this asana, the practitioner's spine naturally straightens. This is useful for people who have sciatica or sacral infections (S, 2008). It stimulates digestion process. This helps in proper movement of apana in downward position resulting in healthy bowel movement.
- Tadasana 1 : This creates a sense of equilibrium. The body is stretched here, and the whole spinal column loosens from top to bottom. The organs and muscles of the abdomen are massaged and toned (S, 2008).
- Trikonasana series: For this study only trikonasana and parvakonasana are selected from the trikonasana series. These konasanas create strong influence on the region of waist. The entire nervous system, especially the spinal nerves, is toned, and muscles and joints are loosened, revitalising the entire body (S, 2008).

- Pascimottanasana: Forward bend during this asana creates contraction of abdomen. Classical benefits of Hathapradipika says that by the practice of this asana one can overcome obesity. By doing this, one will attain fitness and become disease-free (S, 2008) [26].This asana tones all of the abdominal organs, as well as the liver, pancreas, kidneys, and adrenal gland, and helps in the reduction of diabetes, flatulence, and constipation. By massaging the pelvic area, this procedure helps to relieve a number of sexual ailments. As a result, this practise will also help to alleviate the effects of menstrual disorder. This is one of the most effective techniques for balancing the nervous and pranic energies in the body.
- Purvottanasana: It is the counter pose for pascimottanasana that also can be practiced individually. It extends the spine and spinal muscles. It removes strain felt during pascimottanasana.
- Pavanamuktasana series: This study involves pavanamuktasana, bhujangasana, salabhasana and dhaurasana from pavanamuktasana series. All these asanas help efficiently in removing problems related to spine, respiratory and digestive systems. As the name suggests pavana means air or vayu is regulated by this practice by improving peristaltic movement facilitating healthy bowel movement. Indigestion, flatulence and constipation can be relieved by these series. Bhujangasana helps to improve lung capacity by expansion of chest area and can be helpful in reducing respiratory disorders. Dhanurasana gives massaging effect to abdominal organs and digestion capacity is improved by this practice. In the case of oligomenorrhea, Dhanurasana strengthens the uterus while also increasing blood flow and relieving back pain during menstruation. It even stretches the muscles in the back of the trunk and the groin (Digambaraji, 1998) [27].
- Janusirsana: This asana has similar benefits to pascimottanasana (Prabhu, Effect of yogasanas on menstrual cramps in young adult females with primary dysmenorrhea, 2019).The heel pushes against the perineum, activating the organs associated with the urinary and reproductive systems. This procedure

extends the pelvic region and relieves painful bleeding by enhancing pelvic circulation.
- Mahamudra: Scriptural references says that it must be practiced by adopting bandha and kumbhakas . This practise can also be used to treat diseases like tuberculosis, constipation/piles, glandular enlargement, indigestion, and skin diseases like leprosy (S, 2008).
- Upavistakonasana & Baddhakonasana: By lifting the uterus upward, Baddhakonasana relieves uterine congestion. Menstrual flow becomes more normal as a result of this. Upavistakonasana is a great way to alleviate dysmenorrhea (K, 1998).
- Bharadwajasana: This practice gives sufficient twist to sides of abdominal regions.The pelvic area is extended or enlarged, resulting in proper massage of internal organs or the pancreas, as well as increased blood flow to the uterine region. It assists in the treatment of diabetes by encouraging the pancreas to secrete more insulin. The relief of congestion in the pelvic area also helps to alleviate pain during menses.
- Viparitakarani: It is one of the best practice. Hathapradipika explains all the benefits of viparitakarani as regular practice improves gastric fire and therefore one must consume ample food. After six months of regular practice wrinkles on the body and grey hair disappear and also delays aging process (K, 1998). This improves metabolic function that enables proper endocrine function in females with menstrual disorder.
- Halasana and Suptakonasana: These give the abdomen and reproductive organs a contraction effect these endocrine glands are activated, and proper hormone secretion occurs, which aids in the relief of numerous menstrual disorders. Suptakonasana extends the pelvic region, allowing adequate oxygenation of the uterus and urinary organs.

3.2.4 Pranayama:

Pranayama refers to regulation of breath. It is the coordination of prana and citta that helps the mind to work properly. Hathapradipika says, चलेवातेचलंचित्तंनिश्चलेनिश्चलंभवेत् (Digambaraji, 1998). When breathing ceases, the mind remains still, and when breathing stops, the mind becomes still as well. Pranayama is needed for the purification of nadis, which become clogged with impurities over time.It is impossible to progress in one's practise without first purifying these nadis. Pranayama, when done correctly and on a daily basis, can cure any disease. Good outcomes follow appropriate practise. The nadis become purified as breathing becomes slower and deeper and kumbhaka is performed. This results in slimness of the body, lustre on face, clarity of voice, endocrine and gastric secretions are regulated and good health is achieved.

3.2.5 Physiological contributions of Pranayama:

Pranayama comes in a variety of forms, each with its own breathing pattern and physiological, psychological, and biochemical effects. The respiratory rate is slowed as oxygen is drawn in and the outflow of breath is reduced during Pranayama. As a result, metabolic rate decreases and cell relaxation occurs. The respiratory rate, which is usually about 14 to 18 beats per minute, is reduced to 2-3 beats per minute, the entire system hibernates, micro wear-and-tear is slowed, and cells are refreshed (K, 1998). Pranayama that are helpful for decreasing symptoms of menstrual disorders are briefed:

- Ujjayi: According to classical references, Ujjayi practise purifies the nadis and eliminates all nadi diseases such as dropsy and dhatus (K, 1998). Ujjayi relieves congestion in the throat (Digambaraji, 1998) and aid in the proper functioning of the diaphragm It aids in the treatment of insomnia as well as the alleviation of symptoms associated with nervousness and chronic stress (S, Yoga and Kriya, 2008).

- Anuloma-viloma: By the practice of this Pranayama, adequate supply of oxygen is given to the entire body. In addition, carbon dioxide is effectively removed. This practise aids in the removal of nadi congestion and facilitates the flow of prana. By controlling the flow of prana in the body, this induces mental calmness (S, 2008).

- Bhastrika : Classical benefits of Bhastrika expose that this practice cures the diseases of vata, pitta and kapha (S, 2008). And it also aids in the improvement of digestive capability and the revitalization of prana flow. Bhastrika opens up the closed air cells, resulting in increased oxygen transfer and carbon dioxide removal from the body, purifying the lungs (Digambaraji, 1998).
- Bahya kumbhaka: A brief period of hypoxia occurs during this Pranayama. The hormone erthyropoietin, produced by the kidneys in response to hypoxia, stimulates the production of red blood cells in the bone marrow. Erthyropoiesis is the process of red blood cell production (S, 2008) . Hence haemoglobin level in the blood increases and that relieves from anaemic condition.

3.2.6 Dhyana:

It is the stage of culmination of uninterrupted concentration. It induces mental tranquillity (K, 1998). As a consequence, stress is regulated, and hormone harmonisation is possible. Meditation is the cure for the majority of psychiatric and psychosomatic illnesses. The most significant and effective meditational technique is pranava dhyana. It is also called ॐ, Om meditation. Several studies have shown that meditation techniques are useful in decreasing PMS and other symptoms of menstrual disorder.

3.2.7 Relaxation:

Relaxation can be achieved through a number of approaches. This maintains a healthy mix between physical and mental activities. Menstrual disorder relief necessitates both physical and emotional relaxation. Since mental stimulation is needed to relieve physical pain and body disturbances during menstruation. Only by proper relaxation will the pituitary secretions of the HPO axis be balanced, resulting in safe menstruation. Yoganidra and savasana are effective relaxation techniques. Yoganidra practise reduced anxiety and depression in patients with menstrual irregularities (S, 2008).

3.2.8 Appliance of Yoga Therapy :

A protocol for yoga therapy was prepared in view of the above mentioned factors. Protocol was prepared in such a way that, the practices given to the subjects helped in reducing the symptoms such as heavy bleeding in menorrhagia subjects and ensured that the flow in oligomenorrhea subjects along with reducing other associated symptoms of menstrual disorder. These were concentrated according to their case history.

Yoga therapy is given in the following order: Lifestyle, asana, Pranayama, mudra, bandha, dhyana and relaxation. Some instructions to be followed by the yoga therapists are:

- ❖ Practices must be given in a specific sequence.
- ❖ Simple asanas to be taught first and difficult ones are introduced progressively according to level of difficulty.
- ❖ Forcing for perfection must be avoided and practiced up to the capacity of the subject.

5. MATERIALS AND METHODS

5.1 Materials and methods

5.1.1 Place of the study: The present study is done in the department of Human Consciousness and Yogic Sciences, Mangalore University, for the girls residing in the Mangalore University Ladies Hostel, Mangalore city of Dakshina Kannada District, Karnataka State, India. The study was conducted for 3 months which involved 2 months practice and one month follow up.

5.1.2 Selection of sample: Sample were selected on voluntary basis, which comes under non-probability sampling method. 100 subjects with symptoms of menstrual disorder who consented to participate in the study were recruited or considered.

5.1.3 Study design: The current study has 2 groups for the comparison. The subjects were divided into two groups namely experimental group and control group of 50 subjects each. Experimental group was further divided into two groups heavy bleeding group with 27subjects and scanty bleeding subjects with23 subjects. Experimental group was introduced to selected yogic practices. Control group was further divided into two groups heavy bleeding with 31subjects and scanty bleeding with19 subjects. Control group was allowed to continue their normal routine and no any modifications were incorporated to them. Yoga therapy sessions were conducted for six days in a week for the duration of one hour.

5.1.4 Criteria:

> Inclusion criteria:
  - The subjects having symptoms of menstrual disorder like irregular menstruation associated with pain and scanty menstruation, mood swings, headache, fatigue will be included.
  - The subjects of age 18-25 years will be included.

> Exclusion criteria:
  - The subjects discharging clots with pathological conditions will be excluded.

- Subjects having Haemoglobin less than 8 g/dl will be excluded.
- Subjects under medication will be excluded.

5.1.5 **Ethical clearance:** The study designs of the present study were approved by the Institutional Human Ethical Committee(IHEC) of Mangalore University.

5.1.6 **Consent:** A written consent was obtained from all the subjects after explaining all details about the present study including purpose of the study, collection of samples, data collection, application of yoga therapy and duration.

5.1.7 **Case history recording:** Detailed case histories of all the subjects were taken systematically and maintained carefully. Many aspects like, history of present illness, history, family history, physical examinations like, sleep, appetite, micturition, bowel were noted. Blood pressure, weight and height were recorded. Blood pressure using sphygmomanometer and weight is determined using weighting machine.

5.1.8 **Medical assessment:** The selection of the subjects and the assessment of the clinical condition were done under the guidance of medical field expert.

5.1.9 **Collection of blood sample:** The blood tests of the subjects were done in a standardized clinical laboratory for the various parameters before and after the study.

5.1.10 **Parameters:**

- ❖ Estrogen (Estradiol) test
- ❖ Luteinizing Hormone test
- ❖ Haemoglobin

- Estrogen (Estradiol) test: An estradiol test is a simple blood test to measure the amount of estradiol in a person's blood. Estradiol, also known as E2, is one of the four types of estrogen that the ovaries chiefly produce. The adrenal glands, placenta, testes, and some tissues also produce smaller amounts of this hormone [15].This test is suggested if one is having following symptoms: Abnormal menstrual periods, abnormal vaginal bleeding, infertility in women, Menopause symptoms [16].

- Luteinizing Hormone test: Luteinizing hormone (LH) is produced in the pituitary gland and is also known as a gonadotropin, and it affects the sex organs in both men and women. For women, it affects ovaries [17]. It plays a role in puberty, menstruation, and fertility. It is tested when a woman is having difficulty getting pregnant, having irregular or absent menstrual periods etc.
- Haemoglobin: Red blood cells carry oxygen around the body using a particular protein called haemoglobin. The haemoglobin test measures the amount of haemoglobin in the red blood. Anaemia is a deficiency caused by decrease of red blood cells in the body. Due to heavy bleeding during periods there is chance of the occurrence of anaemia.

Women: Age > 18years: 12.1 – 15.1 g/dl(Normal range)

5.2 Hypothesis:

- There will be normalisation of level of estrogen and LH in the experimental group subjects after yoga therapy.
- There will be increase of Haemoglobin level in experiment group subjects.
- There will be reduction of symptoms of menstrual disorder and improvement of quality of life in experimental group subjects after yoga therapy.

5.3 Yoga therapy:

A yoga protocol was prepared by considering the condition of the subjects by studying the detailed case history and was validated by the subject expert. The yoga protocol was prepared to improve metabolic activity and to improve the functioning of endocrine glands so that there will be normalisation of hormones in the blood stream. The yogic practices were introduced to the experimental group subjects gradually and individual attention was given during the session. The yogic practices were taught to the subjects six days per week for one month for a period of 2 months.

The following techniques were introduced to the experimental group.

5.3.1 Life Style:

Menstrual problems can be managed in large part by changing one's lifestyle. Most of the factors affecting individual health and quality of life are linked to one's lifestyle.. Life style comprises each and every activity that one does including the intake offood and sleep.Yoga emphasises a proper and safe lifestyle, which includes achar (healthy activities), vichar (healthy thoughts), ahar (healthy food), and vihar (healthy living) (healthy recreation). Subjects were advised to maintain a healthy lifestyle by slightly modifying their routine like sleep on time and getting up early.

5.3.2 Asana : Depending on the nature of the individual, the relevant yogic practices were taught to the experimental group subjects in three stages as below:

Primary Stage	**Secondary Stage**	**Tertiary Stage**
Svastikasana	Pascimottanasana	Mahamudra
Vajrasana	Shalabhasana,	Upavistakonasana
Supta vajrasana	Dhanurasana,	Baddhakonasana
Tadasana I	Janusirshasana	Viparitakarani
Trikonasana	Bharadwajasana	Halasana
Parsvakonasa		Suptakonasana
Purvothanasana		
Pavanamuktasana		
Bhujangasana		
Uttanapadasana		
Savasana		

5.3.3 Method of practice of Asana :

Subjects were instructed to perform asanas in a way that Vinyasa and Svasocchvasa are synchronised. In the sthiti (final position) of each of the asanas, along with Drsti (direction of eye sight) there was duration of 5 breathings. The asanas were taught progressively one by one. Only the asanas listed in the primary stage were applied in the initial days. After 8-10 days of practice, asanas listed in the secondary stage were progressively applied, one by one. Asanas from the third stage were taught once all asanas were practised from the list of primary and secondary by the subjects satisfactorily. All the asanas were applied by observing the condition of the individual.

Sequence of Asana :

Asanas were practised in the series given below :

Svastikasana, Vajrasana, Supta vajrasana, Tadasana I, Trikonasana, Parsvakonasa, Pascimottanasana, Purvothanasana, Pavanamuktasana, Bhujangasana, Shalabhasana, Dhanurasana, Janusirshasana, Mahamudra, Upavistakonasana, Baddhakonasana, Bharadwajasana, , Viparitakarani, Halasana, Suptakonasana, Uttanapadasana Shavasana.

5.3.4 Pranayama:

The series of pranayama incorporated to the experimental group subjects Ujjayi, Anuloma-Viloma, Bhastrika and Bahya Kumbhaka. Only Ujjayi and Anuloma-Viloma were taught to the subjects for the duration of 21 cycles. After 8 10 days of practice, i.e in the second stage, Bhastrika was introduced to the subjects depending on the ability and body condition of the subjects. The subjects practised Bhastrika for 10-12 cycles. Bahya Kumbhaka was taught in the tertiary stage. In the beginning, it was suggested to practice only 5 cycles of Kumbhaka. Later as the subject gets hold over the Kumbhaka practice, the number of cycle was increased gradually up to 10 according to the capability of the subjects. The subjects were observed in every session and guided to practice the pranayama in such a way that the breathings should be slower and deeper.

5.3.5 Dhyana :

Pranava dhyana was taught to most of the subjects and suggested to practice for 6 months. The duration of the dhyana was 12 rounds in the initial days of incorporation. In the secondary stage, the subjects were suggested to practise 24 rounds and 48 rounds in the tertiary stage.

5.3.6 Relaxation :

In the beginning of the asana practice itself, savasana was implemented for the duration of 10 minutes with toe to head observation.

5.4 Statistical Analysis:

For both experimental and control group subjects, haematological parameters were tested in the laboratory and were recorded prior to the therapy and also after the therapy in pursuance of effect of yoga therapy. The variation in the pre and post values detected reflects the effect of yoga therapy. To distinguish whether the difference in the experimental and control groups are equal statistical tests were performed.

To determine the effect of yoga therapy on quality of life, some parameters like appetite, sleep, bowel and weight were recorded before and after the therapy. Only for the experimental group these observations were recorded. The differences of pre and post values observed express the effect of yoga therapy. Statistical analysis was done by paired t test under the guidance of statistician.

Pictorial representation of study design:

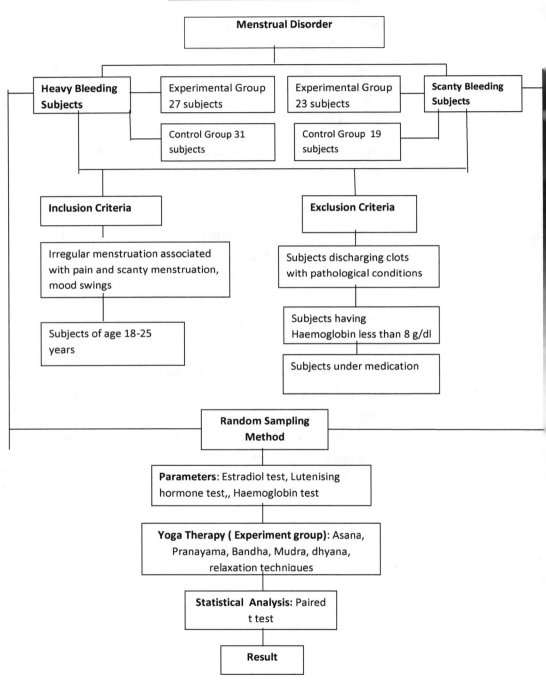

6. RESULTS

In this chapter results of the overall study are described. Here quantification of the results has been done. Result of experimental group is compared with control group by doing the statistical analysis. The data collected for blood tests were analysed using paired 't' test. The level of significance, 'p' is considered as 0.05 to decide the significance of the result. If $p < 0.05$, then the difference is considered statistically significant and non- significant if $p > 0.05$. The difference is considered highly significant if $p < 0.01$. Significant difference of result is found in all the parameters in before and after tests in experimental group subjects when compared to control group.

6.1.1 Demographic Characteristics of the subjects chosen for the study:

Data	Experimental Group	Control Group
Number of subjects	50	50
Range of age	18 – 25 years	18 – 25 years
Marital status	Unmarried	Unmarried
Number of heavy bleeding subjects	27	23
Number of scanty bleeding subjects	31	19

6.1.2 Comparison of pre and post of experimental group subjects:

Sl.No	Parameter	t value	Mean of difference	p value
01.	Estrogen	-1.256	-0.77	0.214
02.	LH	2.815	0.25	0.007
03.	Hb	-8.561	-0.72	2.68E-11

6.1.3 Comparison of pre and post of Control group subjects:

Sl.No	Parameter	t value	Mean of difference	p value
01.	Estrogen	-0.134	-0.05	0.893
02.	LH	-0.614	-0.04	0.541
03.	Hb	0.366	0.01	0.715

Both the groups are further divided into Mennorhagia subjects and Oligomenorrhoea subjects :

6.1.4 Comparison of pre and post test of experimental group of Menorrhagic subjects:

Sl.No	Parameter	t value	Df	Mean of difference	95 percent confidence interval		p value
					Upper	Lower	
01.	Estrogen	2.5803	26	2.44444	0.497105	4.391783	0.01587
02.	LH	-1.995	26	-0.266666	0.54139	0.008061	0.0566
03.	Hb	5.371	26	0.714814	0.441249	0.98838	0.00001266

6.1.5 Comparison of pre and post test of control group of Menorrhagic subjects :

Sl.No	Parameter	t value	Df	Mean of difference	95 percent confidence interval		p value
					Upper	Lower	
01.	Estrogen	0.2436	30	0.1451613	-1.07182	1.362145	0.8092
02.	LH	0.5197	30	0.041935	0.122860	-0.20673	0.6071
03.	Hb	-0.6470	30	-0.025806	-0.107259	0.055646	0.5225

6.1.6 Comparison of experimental and control group: Two sample test.

Sl. No	Parameter	t value	Df	Mean of difference		95 percent confidence interval		p value
				X	Y	Upper	Lower	
01.	Estrogen	-2.109	56	0.14516	2.4444	-4.4829	-0.1155	0.0394
02.	LH	2.0344	56	0.04193	-0.2666	0.00472	0.06124	0.0466
03.	Hb	-5.644	56	-0.0258	0.71481	-1.0034	-0.4777	0.0000054

6.1.7 Comparison of pre and post test of experimental group of Oligomenorrhea subjects :

Sl.No	Parameter	t value	Df	Mean of difference	95 percent confidence interval		p value
					Upper	Lower	
01.	Estrogen	-2.3973	22	-1.195652	-2.2300016	-0.161302	0.02544
02.	LH	-1.9781	22	-0.239130	-0.489839	0.01157389	0.06058
03.	Hb	7.3089	22	0.7391304	0.5294041	0.9488568	0.00000025

6.1.8 Comparison of pre and post test of control group of Oligomenorrhea subjects :

Sl.No	Parameter	t value	Df	Mean of difference	95 percent confidence interval		p value
					Upper	Lower	
01.	Estrogen	-0.73527	18	-0.105263	-0.4060367	0.1955104	0.4716
02.	LH	0.38169	18	0.0157894	-0.0711210	0.10270	0.7072
03.	Hb	0.067335	18	0.0052631	-0.158952	0.1694791	0.9471

6.1.9 Comparison of experimental and control group: Two sample test.

Sl.No	Parameter	t value	Df	Mean of difference		95 percent confidence interval		p value
				X	Y	Upper	Lower	
01.	Estrogen	1.9297	40	-0.1052	-1.19565	-0.05160	2.23285	0.06075
02.	LH	1.841	40	0.01578	-0.23913	-0.02493	0.534778	0.07305
03.	Hb	-5.554	40	0.60526	0.739130	-1.00088	-0.466854	0.0000019

GRAPHICAL REPRESENTATION

6. 12 Comparison of Experimental and Control group

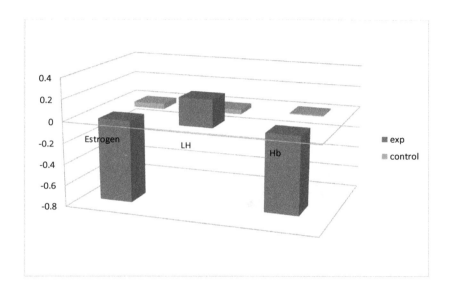

6.13 Distribution of Estrogen, LH & Hb in Menorrhagic subjects

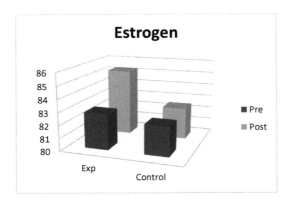

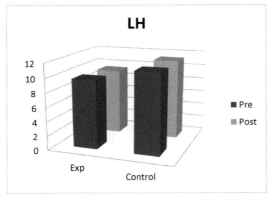

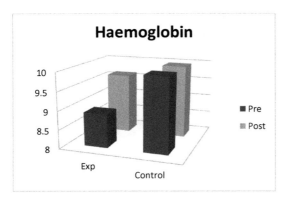

6.14 Distribution of Estrogen, LH & Hb in Oligomenorrhoea subjects

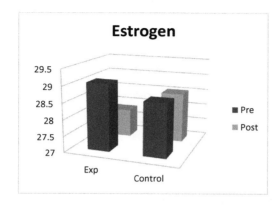

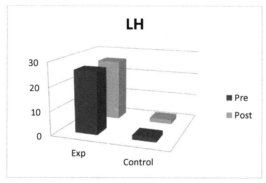

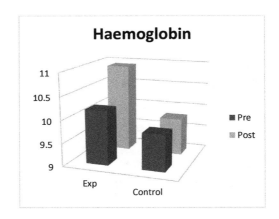

6.15 Comparision of experimental and control group: Menorrhagia

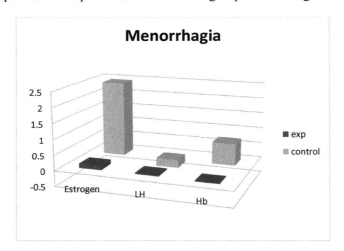

6.16 Comparision of experimental and control group: Oligomenorrhoea

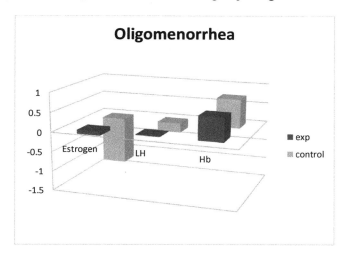

6.10 Summary of effect of yoga on quality of life

	APPETITE n = 21	SLEEP n = 14	BOWEL n = 18	WEIGHT n = 9
Estrogen pre	30.09	23.22	27.90	64.03
Estrogen post	28.86	21.82	26.73	65.52
Luteinising Hormone pre	26.29	20.86	25.16	8.05
Luteinising Hormone post	26.00	20.5	24.82	7.46
Haemoglobin pre	10.22	10.14	10.2	8.61
Haemoglobin post	11.00	10.78	11.00	9.72

6.11 Summary of test results-Quality of life

	APPETITE			SLEEP		
Characters	Mean	t-stat	p-value	Mean	t-stat	p-value
Estrogen	29.48	2.25	0.03	22.52	2.28	0.03
Luteinising Hormone	26.15	2.23	0.037	20.68	2.25	0.04
Haemoglobin	10.61	-7.814	1.67E-07	10.14	-8.003	2.23E-06

	BOWEL			WEIGHT		
Characters	Mean	t-stat	p-value	Mean	t-stat	p-value
Estrogen	27.32	1.984	0.06	64.77	-0.65	0.531
Luteinising Hormone	24.99	2.43	0.026	7.761	6.87	0.00012
Haemoglobin	10.60	-7.055	1.93E-06	9.166	-3.623	0.006

6.17 Graphical representation of quality of life

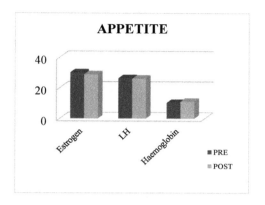

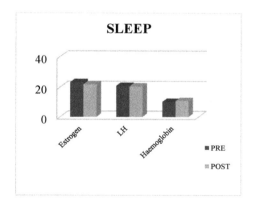

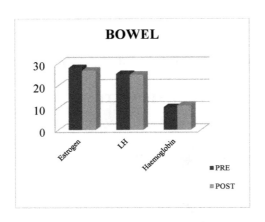

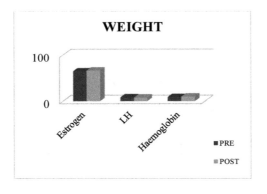

6.2. Discussion:

Total analysis of the data show a remarkable impediment in the experiment group compared to control group across all parameters defined, designating that yoga therapy can produce a positive impact on subjects with heavy bleeding as well as irregular menstruation. Due to unhealthy lifestyle, intake of decreased quality of food, obesity, stress can cause these kinds of menstrual abnormalities. Menstrual cycle indicates the health of a woman. These cycles are maintained by hormones by which when there is imbalance of levels leads to menstrual problems. Due to heavy bleeding during menses there will be reduction of RBC or Haemoglobin count in blood. The result of Haemoglobin count in experimental group clearly shows that there is highly significant role of yoga on increasing the Haemoglobin count.

6.2.1 Estrogen hormone: The test done to measure estrogen level is called estradiol test. The pre and post results of experimental group subjects are compared, mean difference of -0.77 is obtained with p value 0.214 and when pre and post results of control group are compared mean of difference, - 0.05 is obtained with p value 0.893. This result clearly depicts that as a whole, the experimental group attained highly significant result compared to the control group. Both the groups were further divided on the basis of the disorder or the quantity of the bleeding in which the experimental group had 27 menorrhagia (heavy bleeding) subjects and 23 oligomenorrhea(scanty bleeding) subjects and in control group there were 31 menorrhagia subjects and 19 oligomenorrhea subjects.

The mean difference of pre and post results of menorrhagic subjects in the experimental group showed p value 0.01587 and control group subjects showed 0.8092. When this result is compared, it is clear that experimental group subjects received highly significant result but in order to determine whether the difference between these result is statistically significant two- sample test was done and obtained the p value 0.0394 which is evident for the significant result. The mean difference of pre and post results of oligomenorrhea subjects in the experimental group showed p value 0.02544 and control group subjects showed 0.4716. When this result is compared, it is clear that experimental group subjects received highly significant result but in order to determine whether the difference between these result is statistically significant two- sample test was done and obtained the p value 0.06 which states that estradiol test results in oligomenorrhea subjects are less significant when compared to menorrhagia subjects.

6.2.2 Luteinising Hormone: The pre and post results of experimental group subjects are compared, mean difference of 0.25 is obtained with p value 0.007 and when pre and post results of control group are compared mean of difference, - 0. 04 is obtained with p value 0.541. This result clearly depicts that as a whole, the experimental group attained highly significant result compared to the control group. The mean difference of pre and post results of menorrhagic subjects in the experimental group showed p value 0.0566 and control group subjects showed 0.6071. When this result is compared, it is clear that experimental group subjects received highly significant result but in order to determine whether the difference between these result is statistically significant two- sample test was done and obtained the p value 0.0466 which is evident for the significant result. The mean difference of pre and post results of oligomenorrhea subjects in the experimental group showed p value 0.06058 and control group subjects showed 0.7072. When this result is compared, it is clear that experimental group subjects received highly significant result but in order to determine whether the difference between these result is statistically significant two-sample test was done and obtained the p value 0.07305 which states that LH test results in oligomenorrhea subjects are less significant when compared to menorrhagia subjects.

6.2.3 Haemoglobin: The pre and post results of experimental group subjects are compared, mean difference of -0.72 is obtained with p value 2.68E-11 and when pre and post results of control group are compared mean of difference, -0.01 is obtained with p value 0715. This result clearly depicts that as a whole, the experimental group attained highly significant result compared to the control group. The mean difference of pre and post results of menorrhagic subjects in the experimental group showed p value 0.00001 and control group subjects showed 0.5225. When this result is compared, it is clear that experimental group subjects received highly significant result but in order to determine whether the difference between these result is statistically significant two-sample test was done and obtained the p value 0.0000054 which is evident for the significant result. The mean difference of pre and post results of oligomenorrhea subjects in the experimental group showed p value 0.000000025 and control group subjects showed 0.94471. When this result is compared, it is clear that experimental group subjects received highly significant result but in order to determine whether the difference between these result is statistically significant two-sample test was done and obtained the p value 0.00000199 which states that LH test results in both menorrhaia and oligomenorrhea subjects are highly significant.

6.2.4 Assessment of Quality of life:

In order to assess the quality of Life of the subjects of experimental group, the personal history characteristics are considered. In the sample of 50 subjects of experimental group, there were 21 subjects with poor appetite, 14 subjects with sleeplessness, 18 subjects with bowel issues and 9 subjects were underweight. The appetite, bowel, sleep and weight have expressed significant improvement corresponding significant improvement to Estradiol, Luteinising hormone and haemoglobin. By oral discussion with the subjects, it was found that there was improvement in the sleep quality and quantity. They stated that their digestion capacity has improved and were reduction in bowel problem. Subjects also mentioned that there were improvement in their concentration and working capacity. They felt physical and mental relaxation due to the practice of yoga. These results depict the positive impact of yoga on the quality of life of experimental group subjects.

6.2.5 Effect of Yoga Therapy on Anaemic condition of Subjects:

Prior to the yoga therapy there were 18 subjects with menorrhagia had less haemoglobin count. After yoga therapy haemoglobin count of almost all the subjects improved with the significant p value 0.00001.

6.2.6 Impact of Yoga Therapy in reducing symptoms of menstrual disorder:

In the present study there is reduction in symptoms in symptoms such as irregularity of menstruation in experimental group. Subjects having heavy bleeding reported that, after yoga therapy, their complaint have reduced and they did not have to change their sanitary pads frequently like earlier, when sanitary napkins had to change once in every hour or once in every 2 hours. Discomfort and absenteeism in their study place of heavy bleeding subjects during menstruation were also reduced. They felt positive impact on their normal routine and they experienced improvement in their working ability. Heavy bleeding subjects also had issues of decreased Haemoglobin count in blood. By yoga therapy there was improvement in the metabolic activity of the body resulting in more production of RBC and hence Haemoglobin.

Subjects with heavy bleeding reported reduction in their solid discharge, earlier they had excess solid discharge which was painful and unusual. Using sanitary napkins during solid discharge would be troublesome. Because of heavy bleeding, they had sweat formation which reduced post practice. Subjects also reported that they had improved their appetite and reduced fatigue. Changing pads frequently would disturb the sleep pattern. It would increase the tiredness and increase sweating during night. Excess bleeding would also cause vaginal infection such as itching, inflammation and pain. Subjects with scanty bleeding faced problems such as increased weight, increased appetite, social problems also sleep disturbances. Yoga therapy helped these subjects with proper movement in the pelvic region, sufficient supply of oxygen to the cells and hence regularised the bleeding pattern. Appetite was regularised. Some of them had reported burning urination while bleeding before and lot of physical discomfort before yoga therapy. Their metabolism improved which in turn induced proper sleep. The unpredictable flow would cause social problems between people. Post yoga therapy, the bleeding was recognised, the cycle was normalised along with overall consolation. . In previous studies Yoga intervention was found to be associated with reductions in severity of dysmenorrhea and may be effective in lowering serum homocysteine levels after an intervention period of 8 weeks [19], A holistic yoga program for 12 weeks is significantly better than physical exercise in reducing AMH, LH, and testosterone, mFG score for hirsutism, and improving menstrual frequency with non significant changes in body weight, FSH, and prolactin in adolescent PCOS [20]. This is further upheld by the considerable improvement in quality of life in experimental group subjects than in control group subjects. It is proved that yoga therapy have a significant impact in the normalization and regulation of hormonal level (Estrogen and Luteinising hormone) but the rate of success could be depend on the regularity of practice, lifestyle, dietary change and severity of the problem.

7. CONCLUSION

7.1 Conclusion:

Women, as an essential part of society, face a variety of psychological and physiological issues, one of which is menstrual irregularities, which can contribute to infertility, which is a type of dukhah. The only way to overcome this dukhah is to practise yoga regularly and methodically. It is clear that the current study is capable of normalising hormone levels and bringing Haemoglobin levels into an acceptable range. Yoga enhances their quality of life by improving their wellbeing, comfort, and working ability, in addition to eliminating menstrual disorders.

7.2 Limitations of the study:

- The present study could not analyse the significance of yoga on severe conditions of menstrual disorder.
- The study could not assess the changes of hormone levels in different phases of menstrual cycle because of disordered menstruation of subjects.

7.3 Suggestion for the future research

- Future studies can be focussed on a particular phase of menstruation.
- Study can be done by selecting a particular menstrual disorder.
- Study may be undertaken for a longer duration.
- Study can also done with the usage of herbs along with yoga therapy.

APPENDIX

PRACTISING PROCEDURE

SVASTIKĀSANA

- Sit in Samasthithi. i.e keep the legs together and keep the palms on the either side of the thighs near the buttocks. Keep the back straight and looking straightforward breathe for 5 times.
- Exhaling fold the left leg and keep it at the root of the right thigh. Inhale.
- Exhaling fold the right leg and place the right foot over the left ankle. Keep the spine erect. Keep the hands in chin-mudra (keeping the tips of the thumb and fore finger together) over the respective knees. Closing the eyes breathe for 10 times.
- Inhaling stretch the right leg. Exhale there it self.
- Inhaling stretch the left leg.

VAJRĀSANA

- Sit in Samasthiti
- Exhaling fold both the legs together backwards, sit on the heels, place the palms over the respective knees. Looking straight forward breathe for 5 times.
- Inhaling stretch the legs.

SUPTAVAJRĀSANA

- Sit in *Vajrāsana*.
- Exhaling hold the big toes with respective palms from back side.
- Inhaling look upward.
- Exhaling bend forward and place the forehead on the ground. Closing the eyes breathe for 5 times.
- Inhaling come up and release the hands. Exhale
- Inhaling stretch the legs.

SIMHĀSANA

- Sit in *Vajrāsana*. Place the palms on the either side of knee joint.
- Open the mouth extending the tongue out as much as possible. Inhale freely and exhale forcefully through the mouth for 10 times.
- Close the mouth. Sit in *Vajrāsana* position.
- Inhaling stretch the legs.

TADĀSANA I

Stand in samasthithi. i.e.keep the legs together, keep the hands near the thighs. Looking straightforward breathe for 5 times.
- Inhaling slowly lift both the hands, looking upwards join the palms.
- Exhaling slowly bring down the hands.
- Repeat it for 4 more times.

TADASANA II:

- Stand erectly (toes touching each other).
- While inhaling raise the hands and exhaling bend forward.
- Come up while inhaling and exhaling come to step 1.
- Repeat 5 times.

TRIKONĀSANA

- Stand in Samasthithi.
- Inhaling keep the right leg to right side about one leg distance. Simultaneously stretch the hands parallel to the ground.
- Exhaling turn the right foot to right and bend the body to right side. Catch the right big toe by right palm. Looking at the tip of the left hand breathe for 5 times.
- Inhaling come up.
- Exhaling turn the left foot to the left side, bend the body to left and catch the left big toe with left palm. Looking the tip of the right hand breathe for 5 times.

- Inhaling come up.
- Exhaling join the right leg with left leg.

PĀRŚVAKONĀSANA

- Stand in samasthithi.
- Inhaling stretch the right leg to right about one and half leg distance. Simultaneously stretch the hands parallel to the ground.
- Exhaling turn the right foot to right side, bend the right knee joint (about 90^0) and place the right palm on the right side of the right foot on the floor. Stretch the left arm over the left ear. Looking at the tip of the left hand fingers breathe for 5 times.
- Inhaling come up.
- Exhaling turn the left foot to left side, bend the left knee joint (about 90^0) and place the left palm on the left side of the left foot on the floor. Stretch the right arm over the right ear. Looking at the tip of the right hand fingers breathe for 5 times.
- Inhaling come up.
- Exhaling join the right leg with left leg.

PŪRVATĀNĀSANA

- Sit in Samasthithi.
- Inhaling keep the palms about one foot distance backwards. Exhale there its elf.
- Inhaling lift the body on waist by the help of palms and feet. Straighten the arms and legs, stretch the feet in front. Keep the knees and elbows straight. Stretch the neck and leave the head freely back. Closing the eyes breathe for 5 times.
- Exhaling bring down the body. Inhale.
- Exhaling sit in Samasthithi

PAVANAMUKTĀSANA

- Lie down supine on the floor.
- Exhaling bend the right leg and bring it near the chest, interlock the hands over the right knee.
- Inhaling lift the head and touch the forehead to the right knee. Closing the eyes breathe for 5 times.
- Exhaling bring down the head and release the hands.
- Inhaling stretch the right leg.
- Exhaling bend the left leg and bring it near the chest, interlock the hands over the left knee.
- Inhaling lift the head and touch the forehead to the left knee. Closing the eyes breathe for 5 times.
- Exhaling bring down the head and release the hands.
- Inhaling stretch the left leg.
- Exhaling bend both the legs together and bring the knees as near as possible to the chest. Interlock the hands over the knees. Closing the eyes breathe for 5 times.
- Exhaling bring down the head and release the hands.
- Inhaling stretch both legs.

BHUJANGĀSANA

- Lie down on the floor facing downward. Keep the legs together. Keep the palms under the shoulders on the ground.
- Inhaling lift the head and chest without lifting the waist. Bend the head back and look at the middle of the eyebrows. Breathe for 5 times.
- Exhaling slowly come down and release the hands.

ŚALABHĀSANA

- Lie down on the floor facing downward. Place the palms below the respective thighs.
- Press the palms downwards and while inhaling lift the head and legs together. Looking upwards breathe for 5 times.
- Exhaling bring down the legs and head together. Release the hands.

DHANURĀSANA

- Lie down on the floor facing downward.
- Exhaling bend both the legs together, stretch the arms back and hold the ankles with respective hands.
- Inhaling raise the legs, head and chest together, join the ankles. One should stand on the navel region in *sthiti*. Looking upwards breathe for 5 times.
- Exhaling bring down the head and legs.
- Inhaling leave the hands and stretch the legs.

USTRASANA:

- Stand on the knees (as taught)
- Exhaling bend backwards, place the palms on the soles. Close the eyes, breathe 5 times.
- Inhaling come up.

JANUSHIRSHASANA :

- Sit on the ground with stretched legs.
- Exhaling fold the left leg and keep the heel in such a way that it should touch the perineum. Inhale there itself.
- While exhaling hold the right toe, place the forehead on the knee joint. Breathe for 5 times.
- Inhaling release the hands and exhale there itself.
- Inhaling spread the left leg.
- Repeat all the procedures in the other side also

MAHAMUDRA:
- Sit on the ground with stretched legs.
- Exhaling fold the left leg and keep the heel in such a way that it should touch the perineum. Inhale there itself.
- While exhaling bend forward and hold the right toe by both the hands.
- Now slowly raising the head inhale fully. While exhaling slowly bend the neck and hold the breathe outside as long as you can. Inhaling raise your head. Repeat this procedure for 5 times.
- Inhaling release the hands and exhale there itself.
- Inhaling spread the left leg.
- Repeat all the procedures in the other side also.

BHĀRADVĀJĀSANA
- Sit in Samasthiti
- Inhaling fold the left leg backwards and keep left foot by the side of left buttock.
- Exhaling fold the right leg and place the right foot over the left thigh. Inhale.
- Exhaling turn the body fully to right side from the waist and place left palm below the right knee joint on the ground. Hold the right big toe by the right hand from the back side. Looking right back breathe for five times.
- Inhaling turn front and leave the hands. Exhale.
- Inhaling stretch the right leg.
- Exhaling stretch the left leg.
- Repeat the whole procedure for left side.

VIPARĪTAKARANĪ
- Lie down on the floor in supine position. Bring the hands below the thighs.
- Inhaling lift the legs and back by the support of the palms on the buttocks in such a way that the whole body weight should stand on the shoulder and elbows, back should make a slope and legs perpendicular to the ground. Closing the eyes breathe for 25 times.
- Exhaling bring down the body.

UTTĀNAPĀDĀSANA

- Lie down on the floor in supine position.
- Inhaling lift the legs together about 45° from the floor. Exhale.
- Inhaling keep the crown of the head on the ground by the help of palms. Raise the arms and join the palms in front of the knees. Closing the eyes breathe for 5 times.
- Exhaling bring the legs down and keep the head on ground.

UJJAYĪ PRĀNĀYĀMA

- Sit in *Svastikāsana*. Keep the eyes closed and keep the hands in chin-mudra.
- Deeply inhale and completely exhale observing the breathing on the throat for 21 times.

ANULOMA-VILOMA PRĀNĀYĀMA

- Sit in Svastikāsana, keep the left hand in chin-mudra over the left knee and right hand in mrgī-mudra (folding the fore and middle fingers, keeping the other fingers stretched) near the nose. Keep the eyes closed.
- Close the right nostril by the thumb and inhale through the left nostril.
- Close the left nostril by the right ring and small finger, release the thumb, and exhale through the right nostril.
- Inhale through the right nostril.
- Close the right nostril by the thumb, exhale through the left nostril.
  This is one round of Anuloma-Viloma Prānāyāma.
- Practice it for 21 rounds.

BHASTRIKĀ PRĀNĀYĀMA

- Sit in Svastikāsana. Place the palms facing inwards above the respective knees.
- Deeply inhale and forcefully exhale through the nostrils by giving jerks in such a way that complete exhalation felt in the chest, throat and skull.
- Practice it for 10 rounds.

ŚAVĀSANA I

- Lie down on the floor in supine position.
- Keep the right palm over the abdomen and left palm over the chest. Observe the breathing for 5 minutes.

ŚAVĀSANA II

- Lie down on the floor in supine position.
- Keep the hands on the ground (palms facing upwards). Start relaxing from the body parts from toe onwards part by part up to the head. Relax there itself for 5 minutes.

YOGANIDRĀ

I. **Preparation** : Lie down on the floor in supine position.

Spread the legs and hands (palms facing upwards), close the eyes. Keep the body in a relaxed state.

Deeply inhale, exhale completely .... (3 times).

II. **Resolve** : Take a firm decision oneself "I am aware ....

I am going to practice yoganidra ...."

Say it for 3 times (pause).

III. **Practice** : Observe the body parts

1. **Right side** : Right hand, right hand fingers, thumb, second finger, third finger, fourth finger, fifth finger, palm of the hand, back of the hand, the wrist, the lower arm, the elbow, the shoulder, the right chest, the right abdomen, the right waist, the right hip, the right thigh, the knee joint, the calf muscle, the ankle, the heel, the sole, the big toe, second toe, third toe, fourth toe, fifth toe.

2. **Left side**: Left hand, left hand fingers, thumb, second finger, third finger, fourth finger, fifth finger, palm of the hand, back of the hand, the wrist, the lower arm, the elbow, the shoulder, the left chest, the left abdomen, the left waist, the left hip, the left thigh, the knee joint, the calf muscle, the ankle, the heel, the sole, the big toe, second toe, third toe, fourth toe, fifth toe.

    Deeply inhale, exhale completely .... (3 times)

3. Throat, chin, the right cheek, the left cheek, the lips, nose, tip of the nose, right nostril, left nostril, the eyes, the right eye, the left eye, the right eyebrow, the left eyebrow, the middle of eyebrows, the ears, the right ear, the left ear, the forehead, head, middle of the head.

    Deeply inhale, exhale completely .... (3 times)

4. **Top to Bottom** : Head, forehead, ears, eyebrows, eyes, nose, lips, cheeks, chin, neck, chest, abdomen, navel, shoulders, elbows, wrists, palms, fingers, navel, waist, hips, thighs, knee joints, calf muscles, ankles, heels, soles, toes.

    Deeply inhale, exhale completely .... (3 times)

5. **Bottom to Top** : Toes, soles, heels, ankles, calf muscles, knee joints, thighs, hips, waist, navel, fingers, palms, wrists, elbows, shoulders, navel, chest, neck, chin, cheeks, lips, nose, eyes, eyebrows, ears, forehead, head.

    Deeply inhale, exhale completely .... (3 times)

6. **Top to Bottom** : Head, forehead, ears, eyebrows, eyes, nose, lips, cheeks, chin, neck, chest, abdomen, navel, shoulders, elbows, wrists, palms, fingers, navel, waist, hips, thighs, knee joints, calf muscles, ankles, heels, soles, toes.

    Deeply inhale, exhale completely .... (3 times)

7. **Counting :** Start counting from 1 to 27 and from 27 to 1.

8. **Bottom to navel :** Toes, soles, heels, ankles, calf muscles, knee joints, thighs, hips, waists, navel.

9. **Navel Counting :** Concentrate the awareness on the movement of navel area (pause). Concentrate on this movement in Synchronization with the breathing (pause). Start counting from 1 to 27 (as taught).

10. **Chest counting :** Concentrate the awareness on the movement of the chest area(pause). Concentrate on this movement in Synchronization with the breathing (pause). Start counting from 27 to 1 (as taught).

11. **Throat counting :** Concentrate the awareness on the throat area(pause). Concentrate on this movement in Synchronization with the breathing (pause). Start counting from 1 to 27 (as taught).

12. **Nose Counting :** Concentrate the awareness on the tip of the nose (pause). Concentrate on the tip of the nose in Synchronization with the breathing (pause). Start counting from 27 to 1 (as taught).

13. **Image Visualization :** Imagine that you are standing in front of the prayer hall (pause), go slowly inside (pause), observe the light, concentrate on the light, observe the brightness of the light, concentrate on the brightness of the light(pause),………(about 5 minutes)
Slowly come out from the prayer hall.

14. **Finish :** Draw the mind outside and become aware of the breathing, become aware of the whole body parts, from top to Bottom, become aware of the floor, the room, join the legs, bring close the hands, slowly open the eyes ……….. (stay for 1 minute), get up slowly.

CPSIA information can be obtained
at www.ICGtesting.com
Printed in the USA
BVHW031538091222
653840BV00010B/1190